D0509488

DYNAMIC LIVING

How to Take Charge
of Your Health

Aileen Ludington, MD

Hans Diehl, DrHSc, MPH

Lawson Dumbeck, MEd

Review and Herald® Publishing Association
55 West Oak Ridge Drive
Hagerstown, MD 21740

Caution:

The information in this book is not intended to replace medical advice or treatment. Questions about symptoms and medications, general or specific, should be addressed to your physician.

Table of Contents

Introduction
    About This Book 5

Health Outlook
    1. Balance 6
    2. Costs...8
    3. Western Diet.....................................10
    4. Nutrition..12
    5. Children 14
    6. Aging..16

Lifestyle Diseases
    7. Heart Disease 18
    8. Reversing Heart Disease 20
    9. Hypertension 22
    10. Stroke..24
    11. Cancer..26
    12. Adult Onset Diabetes 28
    13. Osteoporosis.................................30
    14. Obesity 32

Weight Control
    15. Myths and Fads.............................34
    16. Diets..36
    17. Soft Drinks 38
    18. Snacks 40
    19. Exercise..42
    20. Calories 44
    21. Ideal Weight..................................46
    22. Fail-Safe Formula 48

Understanding Food
    23. Starch 50

24. Sugar 52

25. Bread 54

26. Protein...56

27. Milk...58

28. Meat 60

29. Fat 62

30. Cholesterol 64

31. Fiber...66

32. Salt 68

33. Vitamins and Minerals...70

Emotional Health

34. Stress...72

35. Depression 74

36. Emotions 76

37. Mind Power...78

Natural Remedies

38. Plant Food 80

39. Digestion 82

40. Fighting Fads...84

41. Breakfast...86

42. Exercise...88

43. Super Fluid 90

44. Bottled or Tap? 92

45. Sunlight 94

46. Tobacco 96

47. Alcohol 98

48. Caffeine 100

49. Drugs 102

50. Air 104

51. Rest...106

52. Trust in Divine Power 108

Appendix

Testing Your Knowledge...110

Recommended Cookbooks 112

About This Book

This activity-oriented companion to *Dynamic Living* is designed to change lives. It contains recipes, tips, and how-to advice that will guide you to a healthier way of living.

When you have worked through this book, you will possess new skills. You will know how to reduce your risk of heart disease, cancer, diabetes, stroke, and the host of other lifestyle-related diseases that, together, account for eight of the ten leading causes of illness and death in North America.

This workbook is unlike most books on health. It encourages you to become personally involved through an abundance of exercises, activities, and examples. Since real change takes time, it is divided into 52 easy-to-understand units. Work through them at your own pace. One a week is ideal, but you can choose to go as quickly, or as slowly, as you like.

Individual Study:

The workbook, in combination with *Dynamic Living,* provides a complete program of self-study. The information is on the cutting edge of medical science, and the practical, hands-on approach ensures that you can use what you learn immediately.

Workshops and Seminars:

The material in this book can be used as the basis for workshops and seminars. There are sections on nutrition, foods, preventing the killer diseases, weight control, emotional health, and natural remedies. Each unit contains activities and exercises to encourage discussion and motivate participants.

Today, you can do more for your health than any doctor or hospital. This workbook shows you how. Day-by-day and step-by-step.

Unit 1: Balance

Chapter Summary

Too much of a good thing is a bad thing when your health is involved. Common sense and moderation will do more for you than any health fad or miracle cure. Balance is the key to good health—learn to apply it in all areas of your life.

The Case of the Harried Sales Manager

Joe is a sales manager for a telecommunications company. At work he is always busy, talking with customers, motivating his sales team, or writing reports for a demanding boss. The pressure never lets up. For lunch he has a steak and salad if there are clients to entertain, or else he grabs a double-cheeseburger and fries at a nearby fast-food restaurant. Sometimes there's no time for lunch at all. By the time Joe gets home at night he's exhausted and cranky. "I feel like a wreck," he admits. "After work all I want is to relax in front of the television. I know I should make some changes, but I'm not sure how to start."

Balance Is Common Sense in Action

Imagine that Joe came to you for advice. What common sense changes might you suggest to help him incorporate the principle of balance in his life?

_____

_____

_____

Joe's Solution

Joe made a couple simple changes in his routine. First, he started bringing his lunch to work instead of eating out every day. Packing a lunch made it easy to eat more fruits, vegetables, and whole-grain foods, and helped him cut down on high-fat, high-calorie, restaurant fare. Second, Joe and his wife, Amy, now take a brisk walk in the evening when he gets home.

When asked if the changes have been worth it, Joe smiles. "I feel more relaxed and energetic. I've lost weight, and the walks Amy and I take together have become something we both look forward to. It's hard to believe the dramatic impact these changes have made in my life."

How About You?

Now that you have seen how Joe has applied the principle of balance in his life, take a moment to examine your own. Is there an area in your life that is out of balance? If so, write it here:

_____

_____

_____

_____

What are some things you could do this week to bring more balance to this part of your life? List your ideas:

_____

_____

_____

_____

This Week:

Balance is the key to a healthful, happy life. This week make a commitment to act on the ideas you have just written down. Make the principle of balance work for you.

Unit 2: Costs

Chapter Summary

The poor health of employees costs business and government billions of dollars each year. Many companies are now encouraging their employees to adopt healthier lifestyles because a healthy workforce helps keep costs down and profits up.

Individuals and Families Save Money Too!

You don't have to own a company to enjoy the financial benefits of good health. Individuals and families find that a healthful lifestyle makes dollars and sense for them, too.

How Staying Well Saves You Money

Lower insurance costs: Some insurance companies offer big discounts on life and private health insurance to individuals who take care of themselves. Look at how much a male, 35-year-old, non-smoker can save on life insurance premiums.

Cost for $100,000 Life Insurance Policy

Healthy American*	Nonsmoker	Smoker
$169	$188	$326

* Healthy American discount applies to people who exercise, reduce salt intake, and use seat belts.

Spend less on "luxuries": Cigarettes, alcoholic beverages, junk food, and soft drinks. Many of us spend thousands of dollars each year gulping, guzzling, and inhaling these "nonfood" substances. By eliminating them, you avoid their harmful effects on your body—and your wallet.

Reduce your grocery bill: A healthy diet, one low in fat and animal products and high in whole foods, is also an economical one. As foods are processed and refined, nutrition goes down while cost goes up.

Good Food Costs Less

Russet Potato	Frozen French Fries	Potato Chips
$0.43/lb.	$ 0.94/lb.	$ 3.52/lb.

Lower the high cost of health care: A heart attack can cost from $40,000 to $100,000. High-blood-pressure medicines run up to $900 a year. Even if insurance pays most of it, lifestyle related illness still costs you plenty. They say a dollar saved is a dollar earned. Taking steps to ensure you stay healthy is one good way to save your dollars.

The Biggest Benefit Isn't Savings

Getting healthy can save you money, but the best benefits aren't financial. They are the ones you can enjoy every day in the form of increased energy, freedom from disease, and a longer, happier life.

This Week:

Instead of snacking on salty, high-fat chips, try this money-saving alternative:

Crisped Tortilla Chips

1 pkg. of 12 corn tortillas   ½ tsp. onion powder
½ tsp. garlic powder

Arrange the tortillas in a stack. Cut the stack into quarters, and then cut each quarter in half. Lay the wedges on nonstick baking sheets. Avoid overlapping the pieces. Sprinkle them with onion and garlic powder (optional). Bake in a preheated, 375-400 degree oven until the chips are crisp.

Unit 3: Western Diet

Chapter Summary

One hundred years ago only a few Americans suffered from heart disease, stroke, and cancer. Today, lifestyle-related illnesses account for the majority of deaths in North America. The good news is that you don't have to become a statistic. By adopting better diet and lifestyle habits, you can live longer and enjoy a healthier, more productive life.

The Choice Is Yours

You can have the same freedom from heart disease, stroke, and cancer that our ancestors enjoyed simply by changing your habits of diet and exercise. It's possible. All you need are the three essentials.

The Three Essentials

Desire: To modify a habit you must want to change. Old patterns are comfortable. To break their grip you need a strong desire to energize you.

Knowledge: Desire alone can't change entrenched lifestyle patterns. You must also know what to change and understand why you should change it.

For instance, although everyone wants to avoid heart disease, achieving this is impossible without a knowledge of the harmful effects of excess cholesterol and fat in the diet.

Skill: Just knowing what to do isn't enough. You need to know how to do it and then practice until the new behavior becomes automatic.

Skills that promote health include things like learning how to cook low-fat meals, developing a program of regular exercise, reading food labels to avoid highly salted products, and becoming skilled at choosing healthful food at restaurants.

The lack of such skills leaves many people struggling when they attempt to make lifestyle changes. New, unfamiliar practices seem like a lot of work, and there is a big temptation to revert back to old, unhealthful ways.

Fortunately, as new patterns take hold they become just as automatic as the old ones once were, but only if practiced regularly over time.

This Week:

To demonstrate how the three essentials can be applied in your life, try a simple experiment. Eat one or two servings of fresh fruit every morning for the next three weeks.

1. Desire: It's probably safe to assume that you have the desire to protect yourself from disease and live a longer, healthier life.

2. Knowledge: All you really need to know is that fruit is high in the vitamins, minerals, and fiber your body needs. It played a big part in the diet that protected people 100 years ago.

3. Skill: You already have the skills you need. After all, what is easier to prepare than fresh fruit?

Take two or three minutes to jot down as many different types of fruit as you can think of. Can you sample them all during the next few weeks?

Your Fresh Fruit List

_____

_____

_____

_____

_____

_____

Unit 4: Nutrition

Chapter Summary
Too much! Too much sugar, refined foods, salt, fat, protein, beverages, and snacks in our diet is a deadly mix. Only by eating less of these substances and eating more whole-plant foods can we enjoy optimum health and energy.

Seven Serious Offenders
Chapter 4 in *Dynamic Living* lists seven problems with the Western diet. In this exercise, write the letter of the correct description in each blank.

___ Sugar   ___ Snacks   ___ Fat   ___ Salt
___ Protein   ___ Beverages   ___ Refined Foods

A. Americans consume these instead of water. Most are loaded with calories and chemicals.

B. The fiber that protects us from certain cancers, stabilizes blood sugar, and controls weight is removed from these foods.

C. North Americans eat up to 20 times more than they need. It contributes to high blood pressure, heart failure, and kidney disease.

D. Many people get 40% of their daily calories from this. It plugs arteries and contributes to overweight and Type 2 diabetes.

E. It makes up about 20% of America's daily calories, yet provides no fiber or nutrients.

F. Americans eat two to three times more of this than they need. Scientists now recognize that too much can be harmful.

G. These often take the place of real food. They are low in nutrition and disrupt digestion.

Americans Have a "Fat Tooth"

As you've noticed, fat is one of the prime offenders in the Western diet. We eat too much of it. About 40% of the calories in the typical diet comes from fat. Research, however, suggests this total should be under 20%.

Americans have a "fat tooth" and they pay for it with heart attacks, strokes, obesity, and other diseases.

Slimming Your Salad Down

One of the best places to cut the fat is on your salad. Too many people take nutritious greens and turn them into a high-fat nightmare by adding thick, oily dressings. Restaurants are notorious for this. At most of them you don't get a little dressing to go with your salad—you get a little salad to go with your dressing.

Next time your waiter hands you a menu, order your salad with a low-calorie dressing on the side. Better yet, ask for lemon wedges and squeeze the juice on yourself. It's a good low-calorie, no-fat alternative.

This Week:

Four tablespoons of Blue Cheese or Ranch dressing adds 300 calories to a salad. That is 300 calories you don't need. This week try your salads with lemon, or mix up some super salad dressing using this recipe.

Super Salad Dressing

¼ c.	water
¼ c.	lemon juice
¼ tsp.	garlic powder
¼ tsp.	Italian seasoning
¼ tsp.	onion salt

Combine all ingredients and shake well. It gets better with age.

Unit 5: Children

Chapter Summary

Hours of television, Nintendo, and the easy availability of high-calorie snacks are creating a generation of super-fat children. Their obesity predisposes them to a host of lifestyle related illnesses, and has been linked to serious psychological problems. Families can help these children by adopting proper eating and lifestyle habits. Good health is a family affair.

Not-So-Little Jimmy

Jimmy is overweight for an 11-year-old. The heaviest child in his class, he is often teased by the other children. Because he sees himself as slow and awkward, he resists participating in physical education and afterschool sports programs. Instead, Jimmy spends his afternoons at home watching television, playing video games, and snacking on pop, chips, and other goodies.

June and George, Jimmy's parents, are learning how lifestyle affects health and well-being. They're making efforts to change their own lifestyle, and also want to help their son. After some discussion, they have come up with three strategies.

1. Lead by Example

Since children learn by example, June and George committed themselves to being better role models. They decided that this means regular exercise and no snacking for either of them.

Could you be a better role model for your children and others in your family? What are some specific things you could do?

_____

_____

_____

2. Create a Supportive Home Environment

To help Jimmy control his snacking, his parents stopped buying soft drinks, chips, and cookies. These high-calorie temptations were replaced with good, old-fashioned fruits and vegetables. Television watching and video games were also limited.

The environment we live in strongly influences what we eat and how we live. Does your home environment help you achieve your lifestyle goals? What could you do to make it better?

_____

_____

_____

3. Involve Family Members

Jimmy was not silent as his life was rearranged, but his howls of protest were tempered by including him in the process. June and George explained the reasons for the changes, and listened carefully to Jimmy's concerns. Together, the three of them chose new recipes to try. In the evening, Jimmy rode his bike while his parents walked or jogged. The changes were difficult at first, but after a time they became routine and, eventually, enjoyed.

People tend to resist changes in those close to them. By explaining why you are making changes and enlisting the aid of others, you can turn resistance into support. How could you involve your children in the lifestyle changes you are making?

_____

_____

_____

This Week:

Use the ideas you came up with in this unit to make your home a place where good eating habits can flourish. Involve your family in the changes.

Unit 6: Aging

Chapter Summary

A diet of rich, refined foods and a lack of exercise can make you old before your time. But with a healthy lifestyle, worthwhile goals, and a positive mental attitude, it is possible to enjoy life well into your golden years.

Super Seniors

At age 66, Hulda Crooks decided to take on a new challenge—mountain climbing. In the 25 years since, she has scaled some of North America's tallest peaks. Recently, she became the oldest woman ever to ascend Mt. Fuji, the tallest mountain in Japan.

Mrs. Crooks is not alone. Newspaper articles recently chronicled the success of an 80-year-old Seattle man. He climbed 14,000 feet to stand on the pinnacle of ice-covered Mt. Rainier.

Not everyone wants to test their endurance on the world's great mountains, but we all want to live productive, useful lives. As you are discovering, a healthful diet and sound lifestyle practices can keep you going strong in your later years. How you treat your body today will influence your health tomorrow and far into the future.

What's in Your Future?

Take a moment to imagine yourself on your 90th birthday. Are you standing atop a mountain? Painting a picture? Celebrating life with family and friends? Or are you ill and isolated?

Research confirms that a positive attitude is important for physical health and happiness. Without purpose, goals, and productive social activities, we age quickly. Do you have interests and goals that will carry you through your lifetime?

In the space below, list three interests or goals you would like to pursue. Is there something you've always wanted to try? Some place you want to visit? Something you hope to contribute? Use your imagination and list them on the lines below.

_____

_____

_____

_____

One Step at a Time

Hulda Crooks didn't get to the top of a mountain by magic: she did it one step at a time. In the previous exercise, you've listed some things you would like to do. Now imagine the first steps you must take to achieve them.

Choose one of the goals you've listed. If you were going to pursue it, what would be the first step you would take? For example, if you wanted to travel you might get brochures from a travel agent or talk to a friend who has taken a similar trip. Big goals are achieved by taking small steps. Write down those first steps for the goal you have chosen in the space below.

_____

_____

_____

_____

This Week:

They say you are as young as you feel. Start feeling younger by taking that first small step toward a meaningful goal. Learning to create your own purpose and goals (rather than relying on work or family responsibilities to create them for you) is one way to ensure healthy and happy senior years.

Unit 7: Heart Disease

Chapter Summary

We are born with clean, flexible arteries, but excessive fat and cholesterol in the diet can clog them. Eventually this chokes off the oxygen supply to vital organs. Most medical treatment is temporary, at best. If we want to stop heart disease from being the number one killer in North America, lifestyle change is the most promising solution.

Seeing Is Believing

The *HeartScreen* test will help you identify and understand your own risk factors, and guide you in dealing with them. It will approximate your relative risk and will help you identify areas that you may want to work on. In this test, eight risk factors are listed, and scores from 1 to 8 are assigned to each factor.

HeartScreen: Interpreting Your Score

0-6 Ideal	Development of heart disease or stroke is extremely unlikely, especially if your cholesterol level is below 180.
7-14 Elevated	The development of heart disease or stroke is about one-third of the U.S. average, yet three times higher than for the Ideal group.
15-22 High	This is the average. You cannot afford to be average because your risk is 10 times higher than the Ideal group.
23-30 Very High Risk	The development of heart disease and stroke is about three times the U.S. average, or 30 times higher than the Ideal group. Action is imperative! You may be able to drop 4-6 points within 4 to 8 weeks by lowering cholesterol and blood pressure through dietary change.
31-38 Danger!	The likelihood of having a heart attack or stroke is about 4 to 6 times the U.S. average and about 50 times higher than the Ideal group. Set goals and take action without delay!

This Week:

If you don't know your cholesterol, triglycerides, and blood pressure, you need to find out. See your physician. The test takes only a few minutes. Make an appointment this week. What you learn can help save your life.

HeartScreen
Self Scoring Test of Heart Attack and Stroke Risk

Risk Level and Score

Risk Factor	0	1	2	3	4	5	6	7	8
1. Cholesterol* (mg %)	under 160	160-179	180-199	200-219	220-239	240-259	260-279	280-299	300 plus
2. Blood Pressure* (mmHg)	under 110	110-119	120-129	130-139	140-159	160 plus			
3. Smoking (cig./day)	none	up to 5	5-9	10-19	20-29	30+			
4. Overweight** (in %)	0-4%	5-9%	10-14%	15-19%	20-29%	30%+			
5. Triglycerides* (mg %)	under 100	100-149	150-249	250-349	350+				
6. Diabetes (duration)	none	under 5 years	5-10 years	10+ years					
7. Resting Pulse beats/min.	under 56	56-62	63-69	70-80	80+				
8. Stress	rarely tense	tense 3x/wk	tense 2-3x/day	tense & rushed	on tran-quilizers				

Risk Factor	Score
Cholesterol	
Blood Pressure	
Smoking	
Overweight	
Triglycerides	
Diabetes	
Pulse	
Stress	
Total Score:	

* To determine your cholesterol, triglycerides, and blood pressure, just see your physician. The blood test is very simple, inexpensive, takes about five minutes, and it will tell you a lot!

** To determine your percentage of overweight, look up your ideal weight (see text, chapter 21) and subtract it from your actual weight. Divide the difference in pounds by your ideal weight and multiply by 100.

Unit 8: Reversing Heart Disease

Chapter Summary

We have known for years that much of heart disease could be prevented; now we know it can be reversed. Dr. Ornish's study found that plaque-filled arteries in patients on very low-fat, vegetarian diets actually began to open up, allowing more blood and oxygen to the heart and other vital organs.

A Killer on the Loose

Heart attacks are the leading cause of death in the United States—and too much fat is the leading cause of heart attacks. It's been said that excess fat is the most harmful element in the Western diet. Isn't it time you reduced the amount you are eating?

Getting the Fat Out

Dr. Ornish showed that lowering the fat in the diet can reverse heart disease. But making the switch isn't always easy. Asking an American to switch to a low-fat diet is like asking a Chinese chef to cook Italian food—it certainly can be done, but it takes some effort and the willingness to learn new habits.

Here are four general strategies you can use to reduce the fat in your diet.

Substitute: Drink skim milk instead of whole milk. Try a bowl of chilled fruit instead of ice cream for dessert. Look for healthful substitutes to the high fat items in your diet such as cheeses, meats, dressings, and oils.

Reduce: Instead of ordering an 8 oz. steak, try a smaller portion with pasta. Instead of a whole piece of pie, take just a sliver. Eating smaller portions of your favorite high-fat foods allows you to savor a few decadent bites while still cutting fat from your diet.

Eliminate: Eliminate as many temptations as possible. If you don't buy it and bring it into the house, you won't eat it when you are tempted.

Eliminating high-fat foods can work wonders. In Dr. Ornish's headline-making study, the subjects that reversed the narrowing in their arteries were those that eliminated meat and high-fat dairy products entirely.

Construct: Processed foods are stuffed with added fat. If you want to regain control over what goes into your body, cook for yourself. Get a good low-fat cookbook and learn how to prepare delicious new dishes. It's the surest way to protect yourself from the deadly effects of too much fat.

Your Turn

List some specific ways you can apply the principles of substitution, reduction, elimination, and construction to your diet:

Substitution: _____

_____

Reduction: _____

_____

Elimination: _____

_____

Construction: _____

_____

This Week:

Choose at least one of the ways you have listed and put it into practice this week.

Unit 9: Hypertension

Chapter Summary

In North America every third adult has high blood pressure. This puts them at risk of heart attack, stroke, and other debilitating diseases. Obesity, narrowed arteries, estrogen, alcohol, and high salt intake all contribute to the problem. Fortunately, most cases of hypertension can be reversed by simple dietary and lifestyle changes.

Five Ways to Eliminate Essential Hypertension

There are several things you can do to prevent, or reverse, hypertension. *Dynamic Living* highlights five of them in chapter 9. What are they?

_____

_____

_____

_____

Getting the Salt Out

We all need to reduce the amount of salt we eat. Don't worry about not getting enough. If you are like most Americans, you eat up to 20 times more than you need. Three culprits are responsible for much of this harmful excess.

The salt shaker: Throw it away. You already get a dangerously high amount of salt from the food you eat. Don't add to the problem by pouring more on top. Your food will seem bland for a few weeks, but your taste buds will soon adjust and you will begin to enjoy the subtle flavors of foods. The day will come when foods you now think of as delicious will taste salty.

Salty snacks: Things like potato chips, pretzels, and salted nuts are so dangerous they should have a Surgeon General's warning on the box: "Warning, salty snacks are linked to hypertension, stroke, and heart disease. Eat at your own risk." If you must snack, use substitutes like carrot sticks and sliced apples.

Fast foods: If we would cut salt intake to 5 grams a day (one teaspoonful), hypertension would virtually disappear. We will never reach that goal, however, until we break the fast-food habit. A McDonald's cheeseburger alone contains 2 grams of salt. And a three-piece chicken dinner from Kentucky Fried Chicken has a whopping 5.6 grams of salt—more than you should eat for an entire day.

Your Battle Plan

A wise general once said, "Know your enemies." Now that you are aware of the three worst culprits, it's time to do something about them. What are you willing to do to cut salt intake to a level your body can handle? Put your plan in writing.

_____

_____

_____

_____

_____

This Week:

Put your battle plan into action. Begin by throwing away the salt shaker (or at least the salt inside it). Use salt-free spice blends, such as Mrs. Dash, to liven up your food instead.

Unit 10: Stroke

Chapter Summary

Stroke is one of the most dreaded and disabling diseases afflicting Westernized countries, but it is not a disease that attacks indiscriminately. In many populations around the world, stroke is virtually unknown. You can reduce your risk by adopting a lifestyle that promotes healthy arteries and low blood pressure.

Getting the Salt Out

Not salting your food is a good way to start protecting yourself from stroke. Unfortunately, only 25 percent of the salt we eat comes from the shaker. Much of the rest is hidden in processed foods and snacks. Here are a few examples:

PROCESSED FOOD	SALT (mg)
Apple Pie (1 slice)	500
Canned Chili and Beans (1 cup)	3,000
Minute Rice (1 cup)	1,000
Wheaties (2 oz)	1,850
Frozen Pasta au gratin (1 cup)	2,750
Potato Chips (7 oz)	3,500
Tomato Sauce (1/2 cup)	1,950
Canned Tomato Soup (1 cup)	2,200
Corned Beef (3 oz)	2,360
Cheese, American (2 slices)	2,050
Kentucky Fried Chicken (3 pieces)	5,600

Are you surprised? Does it seem like just about everything contains enough salt to pickle your insides? Don't despair. By eating an abundance of unrefined foods you automatically cut the sodium (and fat) in your diet. Eat liberally of fresh fruit, vegetables, grains, and other natural foods.

Become a Label Reader

By carefully reading labels, you can select products low in sodium. Watch for words like "salt," "sodium," and "soda," and avoid products in which these terms are listed among the first five ingredients.

You should also be aware of the FDA's new packaging terminology. Under these guidelines, words appearing on a package have very specific meanings.

FDA's Proposed Packaging Guidelines

	Per Serving
Sodium Free	under 5 mg
Very Low Sodium	under 35 mg
Low Sodium	under 140 mg
Reduced Sodium	a 75% decrease

Don't Get Tricked

Which of these products is lower in sodium?

__ Super Snackies: 200 mg. of sodium per serving.

__ Snackeroos: 300 mg. of sodium per serving.

Super Snackies looks like the better choice, right? Well, that depends on how big a serving is. What if Super Snackies has a serving size of two ounces, and Snackeroos has a serving size of four ounces?

The point is that the makers of salty foods often try to hide the fact by providing information based on ridiculously small serving sizes. Don't be fooled—take serving size into account when you buy.

This Week:

Start checking labels when you shop. Look for low-salt, and no-salt alternatives.

Unit 11: Cancer

Chapter Summary

There is a link between lifestyle factors and many cancers. Smoking, obesity, consumption of alcohol, and a diet that is high in animal products and fat account for 70 percent to 80 percent of all cancers. The good news is that we can fight back. Adopting a healthy lifestyle dramatically lowers our risk.

Miracle Cure?

Imagine the announcement of a pill that would make people immune to cancer. It would be the news-story of the decade. People would flock to their doctors for a prescription, and the inventors would be wealthy beyond belief.

No such pill exists, but chapter 11 of *Dynamic Living* lists four things that, taken together, can prevent the majority of adult cancers. What are they?

_____

_____

_____

_____

Moving Toward an Optimal Diet

One of the items on your list should be a very low-fat, low-cholesterol diet. Many studies have shown that such a diet reduces the risk of heart disease, diabetes, stroke, and many types of cancer.

But making lifestyle changes is not as simple as swallowing a pill. It involves learning new habits and skills. For example, cutting the fat and cholesterol in our diet means preparing more meatless dishes.

One sensible way to develop these skills is by designating a day or two each week for vegetarian-style meals. This gives you a chance to experiment with healthful ways of cooking while gradually building up a new repertoire of favorite new recipes.

Moving Toward the *Optimal Diet*

1. *Use whole-grain breads and cereals.* They have the vitamins, minerals, and fiber that products made with refined flour lack.

2. *Enjoy fresh fruit each day.* Eat a variety of fresh fruit.

3. *Eat a wide variety of vegetables.* Dark-green leafy vegetables are essential for the total vegetarian. (One cup of greens contains more calcium than milk.) Yellow vegetables are high in vitamin A.

4. *Use nuts sparingly.* They are high in minerals and vitamins but also contain lots of fat.

5. *Use a wide variety of beans and peas.* They provide protein and fiber and are low in fat.

Good Eating Begins With Good Recipes

A good cookbook is an investment that will repay you many times over. There is no better tool when it comes to changing your eating habits. Get several. See Appendix, page 108, for more information.

This Week:

Become a part-time vegetarian. Set aside at least one day a week for meals without meat and high-fat dairy products. As you become more experienced, gradually increase the number of meat-free meals you eat each week. Working toward the *Optimal Diet* is an important way to protect your health.

Unit 12: Adult Onset Diabetes

Chapter Summary

One in five people in North America develop diabetes at some point in their life, yet this disease can be prevented and even cured. Low fat, both in the diet and on the body, is the secret.

Needless Suffering

Diabetes is a leading cause of new blindness, foot and leg amputations, and hearing impairment. The worst part is that many people suffer needlessly. Here is the formula that can help beat this disease.

How to Beat Diabetes (Type 2)

1. Eat more natural fiber-rich foods, simply prepared, low in fats, grease, and sugar. Freely use whole grain products, tubers and legumes, salads and vegetables, and eat a substantial breakfast daily—a hot multi-grain cereal will curb your appetite for hours and stabilize your blood sugar.

2. Use fresh whole fruits, but not more than three servings a day (if you have diabetes).

3. Avoid refined and processed foods. They are usually high in fat and sugar, and low in fiber.

4. Markedly reduce fats, oils, and grease. If you use animal products, use them lean and very sparingly, more like a condiment. And watch oily and creamy dressings and sauces.

5. Walk briskly each day. Two 30-minute walks every day are ideal to help burn up the extra sugar in your blood.

6. Work with a physician experienced in the effects of dietary therapy to monitor and adjust your insulin need.

Low-fat Checklist

The main villain in adult-onset diabetes is the enormous amount of fat in our diet. One way we can reduce this overabundance is by using less fat, oil, and grease during cooking. How many of the following do you do?

___ Use non-stick (teflon) cookware to minimize the amount of oil needed to keep food from sticking.

___ Cook onions, green peppers, and other vegetables in broth instead of browning in fat.

___ Use less oil, butter, or fat than a recipe calls for.

___ Eliminate the dabs of butter from casserole toppings and vegetables.

___ Use a nonstick spray or a film of lecithin instead of greasing a casserole dish.

___ Avoid frying.

___ Only cook very lean meat (or better yet, eat no meat at all).

___ Steam or microwave vegetables instead of sautéing them in butter or oil.

What Can You Do?

What steps can you take to reduce the fat in your diet?

_____

_____

_____

_____

_____

This Week:

Make sure you are not adding unnecessary fat and oil to food when you cook. Keeping your meals lean helps keep you lean, too—and that's important if you want to stay free of diabetes.

Unit 13: Osteoporosis

Chapter Summary

Osteoporosis is epidemic in North America, even though the consumption of calcium-rich dairy products and supplements is the highest in the world. By reducing protein intake and adopting a program of daily exercise, the tide can be turned in the battle against this crippling disease.

The Case of the Unsuccessful Savers

Janice and Steve have trouble saving money. Once the bills are paid, there never seems to be any left. After some serious discussion, Janice decided to take a part-time job, and Steve asked his boss for more overtime hours.

What a difference! The next month their paychecks were larger than ever before, but once again there was no money left once the bills were paid. Janice and Steve had increased their spending to match their new income.

Spending Calcium

Something similar happens to people eating a high protein diet. The body "spends" calcium as it processes protein. When there is not enough calcium available in the diet it "borrows" from another source—the bones.

The Western diet provides two or three times the Recommended Daily Allowance of protein. At this level, it is almost impossible to get enough calcium to balance the loss. Slowly over the years the bones become brittle and weak.

The solution is not to take more calcium, but to eat less protein. This allows the body to conserve the calcium already stored in the bones.

High-Calcium, High-Protein Foods

The following chart lists some typical sources of calcium. Notice how high they are in protein. With some of these foods you get a lot of calcium, but you lose even more as the body deals with the excess protein.

Calcium in Concentrated Protein Foods

	Serving Size	Calcium (in mg)	Protein (in gm)
Beef, Chicken	5 oz.	15	34-45
Cheese, Cheddar	4 sl.	900	35
Milk, whole	2 glasses	575	18

High-Calcium, Low-Protein Foods

This chart also lists good sources of calcium. Notice the moderate amounts of protein provided by these foods. An added bonus is that they are all low in fat.

Calcium in Unconcentrated Protein Foods

	Serving size	Calcium (in mg)	Protein (in gm)
Collard greens	1 cup	360	5
Spinach, Broccoli	1 cup	175	5
Bread	2 sl.	50-90	5

Save More Than You Spend

Everyone knows that you can't save money when you spend more than you make. The same principle applies to calcium: You can't keep bones strong if you're flushing the calcium out of them with a high-protein diet.

This Week:

Make an effort to cut down on calcium-robbing, high-protein meats and dairy products. Instead, look to low-protein sources of calcium found in whole grains and dark-green leafy vegetables.

Unit 14: Obesity

Chapter Summary

Being overweight hurts your self-image and lays the foundation for many diseases. The secret of lasting weight loss begins with eating generous amounts of high-fiber foods while limiting animal products and refined foods. Combine this with a brisk, daily walk, and you will easily drop those extra pounds.

Different Problem, Same Cure

Over and over you've heard the same advice: Change your lifestyle to prevent heart disease, stroke, hypertension, diabetes, and a host of other life-shortening diseases.

Why do all these problems have the same solution? Because a low-fat, whole-foods diet is not a gimmick or fad—it's the diet your body was designed for.

It should come as no surprise, then, that the same diet that keeps your arteries clean and reduces the risk of cancer also helps you lose weight—and keep it off for good.

Fats Make Fat

Ounce per ounce the American diet packs a lot of calories. That's because it's high in fat. Look at the comparison: a gram of fat contains more than twice the calories of an equal amount of protein or carbohydrate.

Calories Per Gram	
Fat	9
Alcohol	7
Carbohydrate	4
Protein	4

Count Those Calories

Which of the following contains the most calories: Salties, Vegi-o's, or Yummies?

	Salties	Vegi-o's	Yummies
Carbohydrate	8 g	4 g	2 g
Protein	4 g	5 g	5 g
Fat	2 g	5 g	7 g
	14 g	14 g	14 g

Eat More, Weigh Less

If you picked Yummies, you were correct. Although the serving size was the same for all three, Yummies carries a higher proportion of that weight in fat. As a result, a serving of Yummies contains 91 calories while Vegi-o's has 81 and Salties only 66.

Keep this in mind when you choose your food. You don't have to eat less to cut calories. In fact, if you choose foods that are high in carbohydrates and low in fat, you can eat more than ever and still lose weight. That's good news if you're one of the many who believe going hungry is the only way to get thin.

This Week:

When you shop, check the labels to see how much fat, carbohydrate, and protein the foods you buy contain. Choose those that are high in carbohydrates and low in calorie-dense fats. Remember, if you eat products that carry most of their weight as fat, soon you will be doing the same.

Esau's Pottage

1/3 c. brown rice (raw)	4 c. water
1 c. sautéed onions	1 c. lentils
herbs to taste: marjoram, thyme, Mrs. Dash	

Add ingredients to crockpot and cook until tender. Add herbs shortly before serving. Garnish with parsley and slices of red bell pepper.

Unit 15: Myths and Fads

Chapter Summary

Diets that promise to help you lose weight quickly are suspect. They use tricks that make you weigh less, but often have no lasting effect. Moderately over-weight people can usually lose one to two pounds a week on a well-balanced program of healthy eating and exercise. That's the wise way to take (and keep) weight off.

The Wrong Way to Lose Weight

In chapter 15, *Dynamic Living* lists three wrong ways to lose weight. Look them up, then explain what's wrong with each one.

1. Diuretic (water pill)

2. Protein overdose

3. Very low calorie intake

The Right Way to Lose Weight

Through moderate exercise (walking) and eating a well-balanced diet of low-fat, high-fiber foods, you can lose one to two pounds a week. That might not get you slim in time for summer, but it is a sensible health-conscious approach to long-term weight control.

How Fiber Helps

One of the many virtues of fiber is that it acts as a safety mechanism to keep you from overeating. It helps you feel full before you can eat too many calories.

Fiberless foods lack this automatic shut-off. By the time you feel full, you've eaten enough calories for a family of five. Willpower is the only thing that stands between you and obesity—and we all know how effective that is.

Low-Fiber Foods

All animal products lack fiber. That includes meat, milk, eggs, and cheese.

Processing mills and refines the fiber out of many other foods as well. Sugar, white flour, oils, and most packaged foods fall into this category.

Corn oil is a good example of this process. It takes 14 ears of corn to make one tablespoon of oil. Imagine trying to eat 14 ears of corn at one sitting. Impossible! Yet it's easy to sit down and eat many tablespoons of oil in the form of salad dressings or margarine.

This Week:

Fruits, vegetables, whole grains, and legumes are high in fiber. Eat them in abundance. Start with this low-fat, high-fiber soup. Serve it with hearty whole-wheat bread and a salad. Eat all you want. You'll fill up long before you fatten up.

Split Pea Soup (serves 6)

1 c. split peas	6 c. water
1 c. sautéed onions	¼ c. barley
1 bay leaf	1 potato, chopped
½ tsp. thyme	1 carrot, chopped
1 celery stalk, chopped	½ tbs. sweet basil

Add peas, water, onions, barley, and bay leaf to crockpot and cook until "almost" tender. Add remaining ingredients and cook another 45-60 minutes. Add water if necessary. Leftovers can be used as a spread for bread or as a topping on baked potatoes.

Unit 16: Diets

Chapter Summary

Diets are quick-fix traps that don't last. Many people skip from one to the next, losing weight now and gaining it back later. This cycle is discouraging, defeating, and often dangerous. A lifetime commitment to good health practices is the only safe path to permanent weight control.

Take the Long-Term Approach

It's virtually impossible to lose weight and keep it off if you don't modify your lifestyle. Diets are a short-term solution to a long-term problem. That is why nearly 95 percent of all dieters regain their lost weight within a year.

Make eating the right foods a permanent part of your daily life. This is the solution to weight control. You can beat the bulge and live a happier, healthier life. Here's how:

Basic Guidelines for Good Eating

Turn to the summary in *Dynamic Living.* There you will find basic principles for a way of eating that will help you lose weight permanently. Read each item carefully, imagining how you could incorporate it into your way of living.

Can You Make the Commitment?

Turn inward for a moment. Can you make a long-term commitment to this style of eating? Are you willing to bypass the seductive offers of diets that claim to "melt the pounds off" in favor of a focus on good health?

Take a few minutes to think it through, then answer the following question: "How do I feel about making a life-long switch to this way of eating?" Be honest with yourself. Give the part of you that wants to eat only chocolate as much of a voice as the part that promises never to eat anything "bad" again. Recognize that each voice is an extreme that exists in all of us. Lasting change happens somewhere in the middle, and it doesn't happen overnight. It is a growth process in which new behaviors and values gradually replace old ones. Answer the question now. Use an extra sheet of paper if necessary.

_____

_____

_____

_____

_____

_____

_____

_____

_____

_____

_____

_____

_____

_____

_____

_____

This Week:

Read pages 200 and 201 of *Dynamic Living* several times this week. Study the 10 principles that make up the *Optimal Diet* until you know them well. Start putting them into practice. The reward is worth every effort.

Unit 17: Soft Drinks

Chapter Summary

North Americans, on average, drink more soft drinks than they do water. That means they are getting a lot of calories but not much nutrition. Drinking calorie-loaded beverages is one sure recipe for gaining weight. Switch to water—it's the slender person's drink of choice.

An Inventory

What are you drinking? Sometimes it's eye-opening to find out. Listed below are some beverages you might consume. Try to estimate how many of each you drink on a typical day. Then, for each type of beverage, multiply the number consumed by the number of calories. Write this in the Totals column. When you're done, add all the totals to get a grand total.

Drink (standard serving)	Calories	Number	Total
Coffee, cream & sugar	75	_____	_____
Orange Juice	110	_____	_____
Soda, Juice, Punch	140	_____	_____
Non-fat milk	90	_____	_____
Whole milk	160	_____	_____
Milk shake	425	_____	_____
Beer	150	_____	_____
Cocktail or mixed drink	150	_____	_____
Mineral water	0	_____	
Water	0	_____	
Total Calories			_____

Drinking It On

It takes 3,500 excess calories to make a pound of fat. Assuming you eat enough to maintain your weight, how many days would it take you to drink on an extra pound?

You can calculate this by dividing 3500 by the number of calories you get from beverages each day. For example, if you drank a beer and two coffees the calculation would be:

Total calories for a beer and two coffees = 300.
3500/300 = 11.6 days

In other words, it would take just under 12 days to add an extra pound of fat. At that rate you could gain 30 pounds a year just from what you drink!

Now it's your turn. Take your grand total from the previous exercise and divide it into 3500 to see how long it takes you to drink an extra pound's worth of calories. Fill in the blanks below.

Number of days to drink 3500 calories

3500 / Calories you drink _____ = _____ days

Water Is the Way to Go

If you are serious about controlling your weight, it would be wise to eliminate those sneaky liquid calories. Stop the sodas, lose the liquor, shelve the shakes. Water is what your body needs and craves.

This Week:

Cut calories by drinking more water and fewer high-calorie beverages. If you don't like the taste of tap water, add a twist of lemon or buy bottled water. The more water you drink, the less likely you are to reach for other beverages. That, alone, will cut calories and help stabilize your weight.

Unit 18: Snacks

Chapter Summary

The calories you get from snacking can add up to an extra meal—a big one at that. Many people are able to control their weight just by kicking the snack habit. You can, too, by eating adequate meals high in complex carbohydrates and fiber. These meals will provide you with steady energy you need to make it from one meal to the next.

Warning: Snacking Can Be Hazardous

Stop for a moment and think of the foods you snack on. Do you reach for a juicy apple, or do you unwrap a candy bar? Do you munch raw vegetables, or tear into a sack of chips? Most people opt for high-sugar, high-fat, high-salt goodies to get them from one meal to the next. The extra pounds they wear testify to their devotion.

If you want to lose weight, you must deal with that snack habit. Here are some hints to help you make the change:

Start With a Good Breakfast

Beating the snack habit begins with a hearty breakfast. It should provide plenty of complex carbohydrates for lasting energy. Let whole-grains, which are high in these carbohydrates, form the core of the meal.

Building a Hearty Breakfast

Cereals—cooked cereal, waffles, low-fat granola
Fresh Fruit—all types, especially citrus and melon
Additional fruit—fresh or frozen
Bread—whole-wheat or multi-grain bread
Protein—tofu, legumes, or a little nut butter

Don't Snack for the Wrong Reasons

People snack for many reasons besides hunger. Some people use it as a way to release stress. Others feel guilty taking a break. To them, eating something is a way to legitimize a needed rest.

Do you snack only when you're hungry, or do you use snacks to meet other needs? Think about this, then write down some of your reasons for snacking.

_____

_____

_____

Watch Out for Triggers

Many habits, snacking included, are linked to signals from your environment. For example, you might get the urge for a candy bar whenever you pass that vending machine at work. Or there might be a certain television commercial that makes you want to open a bag of chips. What triggers your urge to snack?

_____

_____

_____

Develop Alternate Behaviors

How do you fight a snack attack? By doing other things to disrupt the pattern. If you are bogged down in your work and need a boost, go for a quick walk to the corner and back. Drink a glass of water rather than the usual soda. If you must eat something, try a piece of fruit or some raw vegetables.

This Week:

Start your mornings with a hearty breakfast, and skip the mid-morning goodies. Together, these habits will help you look good and feel better.

Unit 19: Exercise

Chapter Summary

A regular exercise program helps you lose weight by boosting your metabolism. This causes you to burn more calories even when you aren't exercising. It also increases your energy and endurance and lifts your spirits. Exercise is a high-yield investment.

Important Information

Read the last two sections of chapter 19 of *Dynamic Living*, then answer these questions:

1. How much time a day should an overweight person spend exercising?

   _____

2. What is the safest and best exercise?

   _____

The answers to these questions are important because together they make up the second element of an effective weight-loss program: exercise.

Fortunately, this program can be gentle. You don't need to pump iron or run marathons. Just get yourself some comfortable walking shoes and step out the front door.

No Time to Exercise

Everyone is rushed these days. Even kids and retirees have full calendars. A half hour of exercise every day can seem like an impossible dream.

Many busy people get their exercise out of the way by getting up a little earlier. Some walk during their lunch hour or at break times. Others like to unwind by walking in the evening after work. Be creative and you will find that there is always time for a high-priority activity like exercise.

There Will Be Days

Of course there will be some days when you can't complete your whole exercise routine. When that happens, shoot for a shorter walk. A jaunt to the end of the street or around the house is better than no exercise at all.

Don't strive for perfection and give up when you don't achieve it. Persistence is far more valuable than perfection when it comes to building a healthful lifestyle.

What are some ways you can fit a walk into your day? Write down your ideas in the space below.

_____

_____

_____

_____

No Pain, No Gain?

Maybe you have heard coaches and other "exercise people" say, "No pain, no gain." Forget that advice. If you are trying to control your weight, you don't want gain, anyway. Walking can provide the physical activity you need and boost your metabolism. Exercise doesn't have to hurt to be good for you.

Share It With a Friend

One of the best things about walking is you don't need to do it alone. Walking with others encourages communication. Many couples find it strengthens their relationship, and friends enjoy a companionship that makes the miles fly by.

This Week:

Make walking a part of each day. Start with just 10 minutes a day, and work up from there. When combined with a proper diet, walking is an effective way to keep your weight under control.

Unit 20: Calories

Chapter Summary

We are not born with our appetites, they are habits we develop. By reeducating ourselves to avoid "caloric bombs" and to enjoy more natural, low-fat foods, we can eat more, feel full, and still lose weight.

How Many Calories Do You Need?

Have you ever wondered how many calories you can eat before your body begins storing the excess as fat? To find out, start by calculating how many calories your body needs to keep you alive over a 24-hour period.

Your Basal Metabolic Rate (BMR for short) is the rate at which your body would burn calories if you decided to lay in bed all day. You can estimate your total by multiplying your weight by 10.

BMR Calories Per Day

Weight _____ x 10 = _____ Calories

Now, if you don't have an exercise program or engage in heavy labor, you burn an amount equal to 30 percent of your BMR calories as activity calories. For example, if your BMR calories totaled 1500, you would burn an additional 450 calories as activity calories. Calculate your activity calories by multiplying your BMR calories by .3.

Daily Activity Calories

BMR Calories _____ x .3 = _____ Calories

The final step is to add your BMR and activity calories to get the number of calories you burn in a day. If you eat more than this amount, your body deposits the excess as fat. If you eat less, your body uses fat from its stores and you lose weight.

Calories You Burn Daily

BMR _____ + Activity _____ = _____ Calories

A Caloric Bomb Disaster

It would be hard to exceed your calorie limit on the Optimal Diet because whole foods are high in fiber and low in fat. But when you start adding fat, watch out! Look what happens to this meal:

Food	Cal.	Added Fat	Cal.	Calories
Lettuce and Tomato Salad	40	+ Roquefort dressing	160	200
Whole-Wheat Bread	65	+ Butter	70	135
Broccoli (½ cup)	35	+ Cream Cheese	130	165
Vegetarian Entrée or Broiled Fish (6½ oz.)	220	+ Tartar Sauce	80	300
Large Baked Potato with salsa	135	+ Hollandaise Sauce	180	315
Skim Milk (1 glass)	90	Whole Milk		160
Baked apple with date and walnut	100	Apple Pie a la mode (⅙)		500
Total calories	**685**	**Total calories**		**1,775**

This Week:

Avoid "caloric bombs." Work to reduce the oils, butters, dressings, and gravies you add to your food. This is the week to shift the scales in your favor!

Unit 21: Ideal Weight

Chapter Summary

Knowing your ideal weight is important. Studies show that people who remain near this target live longer, healthier lives. Find out how close (or far) you are from your ideal weight.

Tale of the Scale

The bathroom scale tells the story of our eating and exercise habits. It can also, for better or worse, predict our health in coming years.

Where Do You Weigh In?

Clinically, people 20 percent or more above their ideal weight are classified as obese. Those 10-19 percent above are referred to as overweight. Anyone who's weight ranges from 9 percent under ideal to 9 percent over is considered normal weight, and those 10 percent or more below ideal are underweight.

How do you rate? Complete this easy exercise to find out. Before you begin, you will need to know your weight. A calculator is handy for calculating percentages.

Calculating Your Ideal Weight

For Men:

1. How many inches over five feet are you? _____

2. Multiply that number by six. _____

3. Add 100 to get your ideal weight. _____

For Women:

1. How many inches over five feet are you? _____

2. Multiply that number by five. _____

3. Add 100 to get your ideal weight. _____

For Women and Men:

Large-boned men and women should multiply their ideal weight by 1.05 to get an ideal weight adjusted for their build.

Normal Weight

Multiply your ideal weight by 1.09 = _____

If your weight is below this number, you are in the safe range. Regular exercise and a healthy diet will boost your energy and endurance while keeping your weight stable.

Overweight

Multiply your ideal weight by 1.20 = _____

If your weight is below this number, but above normal weight, you are classified as overweight. Your weight has reached a level where it can affect your health and self-image. It is important to take action now to get your weight under control. Make daily exercise and the Optimal Diet a priority.

Obese

If your weight takes you past overweight then stop! You are in danger and need to take immediate action. Don't let anything stand between you and daily exercise. Learn to cook healthy meals and put the principles learned in the last seven chapters into action. If you change your lifestyle now, you can feel years younger and enjoy a longer, healthier life.

This Week:

A support network can keep you going when you feel like giving up. Find someone else interested in losing weight. Working together will make reaching your goals twice as easy—and twice as enjoyable.

Unit 22: Fail-Safe Formula

Chapter Summary

It is possible to eat as much as you want and still lose weight. The secret is knowing which foods to eat and which to avoid. The whole plant foods that promote good health and prevent disease are also ideal for taking weight off and keeping it off—for good.

Unit Review

Chapter 22 is the last of nine units devoted to weight control. As you have worked through them, we have encouraged you to try many new behaviors. Now that you have had a chance to experiment, we hope you will make them a permanent part of your life. Here they are in review:

Eight Steps to Permanent Weight Control

1. Read labels carefully and choose foods low in fat and refined products.

2. Build your diet around fruits, vegetables, grains, legumes, and other "as grown" foods.

3. Make the *Optimal Diet* (*Dynamic Living*, Summary) your diet.

4. Make water your drink of choice. Avoid high-calorie beverages.

5. Kick the snack habit. Begin each day with a hearty breakfast that makes mid-morning snacking unnecessary.

6. Make exercise a part of your routine. Walk every day.

7. Reduce the oils, butters, dressings, and other fats you add to foods.

8. Develop a support network with others who share your interest in making positive lifestyle changes.

Food Selection

For most of us, getting permanent control of a ballooning waistline requires a radical shift in diet. The table below summarizes the food selection principles presented in *Dynamic Living*.

Eat freely from the following

Fruit: All fresh fruit (avocado and olives sparingly)

Vegetables: All vegetables, greens, herbs, squash

Legumes: All beans, peas, lentils, garbanzos

Tubers: Potatoes, yams, sweet potatoes

Grains: All whole grains, breads, pastas

Nuts: Eat sparingly

— Optional —

Dairy: Nonfat milk, plain yogurt, skim-milk cheeses, buttermilk, and low-fat cottage cheese in moderation.

Eggs: Whites only. Substitute two egg whites for one egg in recipes.

Flesh Foods: *If you insist.* Small amounts (3 oz. no more than three times a week). Skinless fowl, fish fillet, lean beef.

Weight-loss Tips: Attitude

Focus on the hundreds of foods that you can eat, not on those you shouldn't.

Be kind to yourself. It takes time to adapt to a new way of eating and living. Be patient with yourself and don't give up if you make a mistake or slip back into old habits. You are making a long-term investment in yourself. Keep going.

This Week:

This week is a time to integrate everything you have found helpful in the last eight lessons. You can release the thin person inside of you and enjoy a happier, healthier life.

Unit 23: Starch

Chapter Summary

Contrary to what many believe, we need less protein and more starch in our diets. Complex carbohydrates found in fruits, vegetables, and grains provide clean-burning energy and increased endurance. Building your diet around these foods helps keep your arteries clean, your food bill low, and your body healthy.

Naomi's Story

Naomi's mother came back from a doctor's appointment saying, "He told me not to eat any carbohydrates!"

Naomi was concerned. "Mother, you must have misunderstood. Every modern medical doctor knows the body needs carbohydrates. Are you sure he didn't say cholesterol?"

Her mother was uncertain, so they phoned the doctor. Yes, indeed, she had confused cholesterol with carbohydrate. The doctor was happy to explain the difference. "It would have been disastrous," he told them, "to stop eating carbohydrates."

Making Sense of Carbohydrates

Carbohydrate, complex carbohydrate, sugar, starch—it's easy to get confused. The following diagram shows the carbohydrate family tree. Notice how these important energy sources are related.

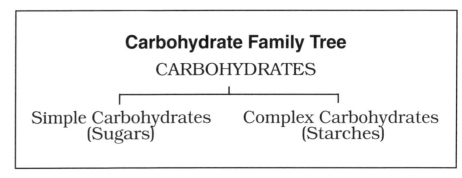

Carbohydrate Family Tree

CARBOHYDRATES

Simple Carbohydrates (Sugars)   Complex Carbohydrates (Starches)

King Potato

The king of the starchy vegetables is the potato. It is filling, nutritious, and tasty. If you have a microwave, it only takes minutes to build a complete meal around this terrific tuber.

Are Potatoes Fattening?

A 5-ounce spud contains only 95 calories. The potato's reputation as a fattening food comes from the way it is served—French fried, baked and slathered with butter or sour cream. It is the added fats, not the potato itself, that are fattening.

Topping Ideas

Lentils: Cook up a pot of lentils with onion and garlic. Ladle them onto a piping hot baked potato. Served with a green salad and whole wheat bread, this meal will satisfy even the heartiest appetite.

Salsa: Ole! It might sound a bit unusual, but salsa makes an excellent topping for a baked potato. It's available at many restaurants. Next time you eat out and the server asks "butter or sour cream?" say, "neither." Ask for salsa instead.

Mrs. Dash Seasoning (salt-free blend): Slice a cooked potato into wedges, sprinkle with Mrs. Dash (the one with the green cap!) seasonings and bake until browned. It's the health-conscious chef's answer to French fries.

Mock Sour-cream: Blenderize low-fat yogurt and cottage cheese, then mix in chopped chives, fresh dill, parsley, green onions, or green pepper.

Leftover soups and stews: There are many wonderful recipes for meatless soups and stews that can do double duty as a topping. Get creative and see what you can come up with.

This Week:

Add more complex carbohydrates to your diet. Enjoy whole-grain foods and potatoes. Complex carbohydrates will fill you up without weighing you down.

Unit 24: Sugar

Chapter Summary

Refined sugars make up around 20 percent of the calories most Americans eat—more than 30 teaspoonfuls per day. Much of this sugar is well hidden in food and beverages. To reduce the sugar in your diet, start by substituting naturally sweet foods for sugared snacks.

Reducing the Sugar in Your Diet

Sugar contains no nutrients or fiber. It is high in calories, and when eaten in excess, it can crowd more nutritious foods out of your diet.

If sugar has a grip on you, here are some simple tips to help you reduce your dependence without eliminating sweet treats altogether.

Reeducate Your Sweet Tooth

A sweet tooth can be reeducated to enjoy less concentrated sweets. Fruit and deserts sweetened with fruit are good alternatives. Try this recipe for a special treat:

Fruit Smoothies

2 frozen, ripe bananas	1 c. pineapple juice
3 or 4 soft dates	2 c. frozen fruit

Blend dates and pineapple juice until smooth. Add bananas and fruit. Blend until it is the consistency of soft ice cream. Delicious! It also makes a great topping for whole-grain waffles and pancakes.

Try these flavors:

strawberries	blueberries
peaches	crushed pineapple
orange juice	fresh blackberries

Indulge Less Frequently

How often do you eat desserts or sweet snacks?

__ 1-4 times/week __ 1-2 times/day

__ 3-4 times/day __ More than 4 times/day

If you answered more than once a day you would benefit from reserving treats for special times.

Eat Smaller Servings

When you do eat sweets and sugared foods, learn to savor small portions. Eat slowly, and make your portion last. You can train yourself to be satisfied with a smaller serving.

Make the Low-Sugar Choice

Choose low-sugar alternatives when shopping. It's not always easy to tell how much sugar a product contains because sugar can be disguised as fructose, sucrose, corn syrup, and other ingredients. When possible, however, buy products that you know are low in sugar.

Your Turn

Think of some ways you can reduce the amount of sugar you are eating. List them below.

_____

_____

_____

_____

_____

This Week:

Try a fruit smoothie. Also, observe how many sweets and other sugary foods you are eating. Use the suggestions in this unit and those you listed on your own to cut back to a healthy level.

Unit 25: Bread

Chapter Summary

During the milling process wheat loses most of its nutrients and fiber. That's why it is important to shop for 100% whole-wheat bread. It is better balanced and more nutritious than white bread.

Look Past the Hype

No bread is all bad, and the makers of even the least nutritious loaves capitalize on this. The wrappers boldly proclaim "Wholesome Goodness," "Natural," and "Fiber." The words and pictures are designed to make you believe you are doing your body a favor by choosing their bread.

Take a Closer Look

Below are the ingredient lists from three loaves of bread. Which one would you choose for optimum nutrition?

1—Whole cracked wheat, unbleached enriched wheat flour [flour, malted barley flour, reduced iron, niacin, thiamin mononitrate, riboflavin], water, honey, raisin syrup, salt, butter, ground raisins, unprocessed millers bran, partially hydrogenated soybean oil, yeast, wheat gluten, wheat germ, vinegar, lecithin.

2—Stone ground whole-wheat flour, multi-grain cereal (rolled oats, rye, cornmeal, sunflower seeds, flax seeds, wheat germ, soy flour), honey, canola oil, yeast, sea salt, vinegar.

3—Enriched bleached flour [barley malt, iron, niacin, thiamine mononitrate, Riboflavin] water, corn syrup, soybean oil, yeast, salt, corn flour, whey, soy flour, cornstarch, nonfat milk, fungal enzymes, ammonia chloride, calcium sulfate, potassium bromate, mono- and diglycerides.

Which loaf would you pick? _____

Did You Make the Best Choice?

Loaf 1: This loaf isn't bad. The first ingredient is whole cracked wheat. Its second ingredient, however, is enriched wheat flour—white flour. It lacks most of the vitamins and fiber of whole-grain flour.

Loaf 2: This is the best choice. Its first ingredient is whole wheat flour. Its second ingredient is seven-grain cereal, which adds the nutrition of a variety of whole grains to the loaf. This loaf feels heavier and more dense than the others.

Loaf 3: This is a loaf of spongy white bread. It lacks vitamins and fiber. Not the best choice for the health-conscious shopper.

This Week:

Look for whole-grain breads when you shop. Read the labels carefully, and don't be mislead by packaging that tries to pass off the "stuff of lies" as the "staff of life."

Delicious Fruit Spreads

Try these delicious toppings on whole-grain toast.

Strawberry Spread

    1 c. strawberries   1 c. mashed, ripe banana

Blend ingredients in a blender until smooth. Heat to a boil in a saucepan, then simmer until the mixture thickens. Stir frequently.

Apple Butter

    1 c. applesauce

Heat ingredients to a boil. Turn heat to low and simmer. Stir frequently until mixture reaches the desired thickness.

Date Butter

    1 c. pitted dates chopped fine   ½ c. water

Boil for 6-8 minutes, stirring until smooth.

Unit 26: Protein

Chapter Summary

Most North Americans eat two or three times more protein than recommended. This excess has been linked to such problems as kidney disease, gout, and osteoporosis. Large quantities of meat and dairy products are not needed—vegetable sources can easily provide your body with all the protein it needs.

The Protein Myth

What kind of foods come to mind when you hear the word protein? Beef? Eggs? Milk? Cheese? Advertisers spend millions each year making certain we feel these foods are indispensable for good health.

The fact is that animal products are not necessary in the human diet. People may choose to eat them for reasons of flavor, habit, and convenience, but nobody should feel they must eat them to get enough protein or nutrients.

High Protein Equals High Fat

Look again at the table in chapter 26 of *Dynamic Living*. As you can see, traditional "high-protein" foods are extremely high in fat. The *Optimal Diet* suggests that less than 20 percent of calories come from fat. Obviously, these foods fail the test.

Plant Protein

All the protein you need is available from plant sources. The following table lists just a few examples.

Notice that, unlike animal products, these sources are naturally low in fat. If you eat a variety of grains, legumes, and vegetables, your diet will never lack the protein your body needs for optimal performance and well-being.

Food Composition as Percent of Total Calories

	Protein	Fat	Carbohydrate
Pinto beans	26	3	71
Lentils	29	3	68
Broccoli	48	9	43
Cabbage	22	7	71
Zucchini	28	5	67
Carrots	10	4	86
Potato	11	1	88
Rice, brown	8	4	88
Wheat flour	16	5	79
Oranges	8	4	88
Peaches	6	2	93

What Are You Eating?

Do you eat all the foods listed above, or do you limit yourself to just a few? Which ones don't you usually eat? List them below.

_____   _____

_____   _____

This Week:

Stretch the boundaries of your diet by sampling some of the foods you have listed. Experiment with the wide variety of tastes and textures available.

Easy Zucchini

6 small zucchinis	3 c. tomato juice
¼ tsp. thyme	½ tsp. Mrs. Dash

Slice zucchini into 1/4-inch thick slices. Place them into baking dish with other ingredients. Cover and bake at 375 degrees for 20 minutes.

Unit 27: Milk

Chapter Summary

Milk is a fine food for babies, but most adults could do without the excess fat, cholesterol, and protein it contains. Fifty percent of whole milk's calories come from fat. Even 2% lowfat milk gets 30% of its calories from fat. For those who wish to use milk, nonfat is preferable.

The *Optimal Diet*

Research on nutrition has clearly demonstrated a unitary dietary principle in dealing with the western killer diseases. In other words, there isn't one diet for treating heart disease, and another for overweight, and yet another for hypertension.

Instead, there is one *Optimal Diet* consisting of a wide variety of plant foods, freely eaten "as grown," prepared with sparing use of fats, oils, sugars, and salt, and almost devoid of refined or processed foods. If animal products are eaten, they are used like a seasoning and not as the focus of the meal.

The following chart compares the typical western diet with the *Optimal Diet*.

Diet Composition

Diet Constituent	U.S. Diet	*Optimal Diet*
Fats and Oils	35-40%	15%
Complex Carbohyd.	22%	60-70%
Refined Sugar	20%	minimal
Cholesterol/day	400 mg	under 50 mg
Salt/day	12-15 gm	under 5 gm
Fiber/day	10 gm	up to 40 gm
Water (Fluids)/day		8 glasses

Does Milk Have a Role in the *Optimal Diet*?

Milk can be a part of the *Optimal Diet*, but it is optional. Many people around the world prosper without it. Based upon what you have learned about milk and the *Optimal Diet,* answer these questions:

Is the use of whole milk in keeping with the *Optimal Diet?* Why or why not?

_____

_____

Is the use of 2% milk in keeping with the *Optimal Diet?* Why or why not?

_____

_____

Is the use of nonfat milk in keeping with the *Optimal Diet?* Why or why not?

_____

_____

Recommendation

Milk is a concentrated protein food and should be used sparingly in nonfat form. Use it in cooking or on cereal if you desire. Soy or tofu milks make good substitutes.

This Week:

Switch to nonfat milk as you shift your eating habits toward the optimum diet.

Unit 28: Meat

Chapter Summary

The evidence keeps mounting that a diet built around whole-plant foods is superior to a meat-based diet. Meat is high in fat and cholesterol. It also lacks the fiber found in grown foods. In populations around the world, vegetarians have better health, are thinner, and live longer.

Kicking the Meat Habit

Many who have made meat and dairy products the center of their meals feel at a loss when trying to plan a meatless menu. For a while their meals seem incomplete without flesh foods.

You can satisfy your appetite on a meat-free diet. It may take a while to adjust, but eventually this way of eating becomes acceptable, and then preferable. Here is a sample menu to get you started planning delicious meat-free meals:

Sample Menu

Breakfast:

Cooked cereal (7-grain cereal) or cold cereal (shredded wheat, Nutrigrain) with skim milk and ½ of a banana or other fresh fruit sliced on top.

Citrus fruit: orange or grapefruit

3 slices of whole-wheat toast with "mashed" banana topped with pineapple ring or slice of kiwi.

Herbal tea.

Lunch:

2 whole-wheat pita (pocket) breads stuffed with lettuce, sprouts, cucumbers, tomatoes, radishes, and some low-fat cottage cheese.

Split pea soup with pearl barley or rice.

Fresh fruit such as papaya, pear, apple.

Dinner:

Whole-wheat spaghetti and tomato sauce.

Tossed salad with low-calorie Italian dressing.

Slice of bread

For dessert: baked apple (microwaved).

Food Selection

As you are planning a more natural dietary program, build your meals around the food categories listed below.

Selection Suggestions

Optimal Foods

Fruit: All fresh fruit (avocado and olives sparingly).

Vegetables: Vegetables, greens, herbs, and squash.

Legumes: All beans, peas, lentils, garbanzos.

Tubers: Potatoes, yams, sweet potatoes.

Grains: All whole grains, bread, pasta.

Nuts: Eat sparingly only.

Optional Foods—*if you insist.*

Dairy: Nonfat milk, plain yogurt, skim-milk cheeses, buttermilk, and low-fat cottage cheese in moderation.

Eggs: Whites only.

Flesh Foods: Small amounts of skinless fowl, fish fillet, lean beef.

This Week:

After trying out the sample menu in this unit, develop your own one-day menu. Use the guidelines provided. Enjoy!

Unit 29: Fat

Chapter Summary

Excess fat in foods is probably the most damaging component of the Western diet. Reducing the amount of fat we eat is essential. Butter, margarine, cooking and salad oils, meats, cheeses, eggs, and whole milk, all must be limited.

The Old Four Food Groups

Do you remember the Four Food Groups? That model of the "proper" diet issued by the U.S. Department of Agriculture in 1956? We've discovered a lot about nutrition since then. One of the things we've learned is that the emphasis on meat and dairy products made the Four Food Groups high in fat, protein, and cholesterol, and low in fiber. Study after study has linked this diet to increased rates of cancer, heart disease, obesity, and diabetes. Clearly a big change is needed: Enter, The *New* Four Food Groups.

The New Four Food Groups is recommended by the Physicians Committee for Responsible Medicine.

The *New* Four Food Groups

Food Group	Servings Per Day	Serving Size
Whole Grains	5 or more	½ cup of hot cereal; one ounce dry cereal; one slice of bread.
Vegetables	3 or more	One cup raw; ½ cup cooked.
Legumes	2 to 3	½ cup cooked beans; four ounces tofu.
Fruits	3 or more	One medium piece of fruit; ½ cup cooked fruit; ½ cup fruit juice.

Your List

Below are the categories from The New Four Food Groups. Under each heading, list foods from that category that you currently eat or would like to try. Chances are you will find that you already eat many foods from The New Four Food Groups.

Whole Grains

_____

_____

_____

_____

Vegetables

_____

_____

_____

_____

Fruits

_____

_____

_____

_____

Legumes

_____

_____

This Week:

Make the New Four Food Groups the foundation of your diet by eating more of the foods you listed above.

Unit 30: Cholesterol

Chapter Summary

Blood cholesterol level is the most important factor in determining a person's risk for developing cardiovascular disease. A rich diet, one high in fat and animal products, raises cholesterol levels. Fortunately, the opposite is true also; a diet very low in fat and cholesterol, and high in fiber, has been shown to lower blood cholesterol levels as much as 20 to 35 percent in four weeks.

Blood Cholesterol Level

Often there are no physical symptoms of the disease before a heart attack occurs. The best way to assess the risk of heart disease before disaster strikes is by looking at blood cholesterol levels. This is the single most important predictor of heart disease.

Do you know your blood cholesterol level? If you don't, make an appointment with your doctor to find out. The procedure is simple, and more importantly, what you learn could save your life.

What is your blood cholesterol level? _____

Take Aggressive Action

If you don't find yourself inside the safety zone with a blood cholesterol level below 160 mg% (4.1mmol/L), don't despair. It is time to take aggressive action. You can lower your cholesterol level by making important lifestyle changes.

Six Ways to Lower Cholesterol Levels

On the next page are six prescriptions that will help lower your cholesterol level. Put a checkmark by the ones you are already working on. Below each item write ways you might achieve that objective. After you're done, turn to chapter 30 of *Dynamic Living* to see how your answers match.

Eat Less Cholesterol

_____

_____

_____

Eat Less Fat

_____

_____

_____

Lose Excess Weight

_____

_____

_____

Eat More Fiber

_____

_____

_____

Exercise More

_____

_____

_____

Medications (if necessary)

_____

_____

This Week:

   Review your list of things you can do to lower your blood cholesterol level. Act on those strategies this week.

Unit 31: Fiber

Chapter Summary

Fiber plays a crucial role in weight control, diabetes, and digestion. It also helps protect against colon cancer. Eating a variety of unrefined foods is the best way to provide your body with the fiber it needs.

Addition and Subtraction

What did you have for supper last night? List everything you ate:

_____

_____

_____

Now, put a plus sign in front of everything that contained whole grains, vegetables, legumes, or fruit. When you have finished, put a minus sign in front of everything that contained sugar, meat, white flour, milk, butter, oil, fat, eggs, or processed foods. It's OK if you end up with several pluses and minuses in front of a single item.

What It All Means

The principle is simple. For every plus, the food you ate added fiber to your diet. For every minus, a refined food added little, if any. Too many minus signs on your list? Then it's time to make some adjustments to your menu.

The Western Diet

The Western diet is full of minuses when it comes to dietary fiber. First, its focus on meat and other animal products provides a shaky foundation. Any food that comes from an animal has absolutely no fiber. Zero.

Second, about half of the calories in the typical American's diet are empty calories. An empty calorie provides no vitamins, minerals, or fiber.

Empty Calories as a Percent of Total Calories

Sugar 21%
Visible fats and oils 20%
Alcohol 9%

Total Empty Calories........................**50%**

This Week:

Start replacing fiber-free foods with fiber-filled foods in your diet. Begin with this flavorful dish:

Black Beans Over Rice

Beans

1¼	c. black beans	5	c. water
1	clove garlic, minced	½	tsp. salt
1	c. onion, chopped	1	green pepper, chopped
1	onion, peeled and stuck with 3 whole cloves.		

Cook beans in Crockpot until they start to get tender. Add garlic and clove studded onion and salt. Cook one hour more.

Rice

4 c. cooked brown rice (1½ c. uncooked rice)

Salsa

16	oz. can of unsalted, unpeeled tomatoes, drained		
¾	c. diced red onion	2	cloves garlic, minced
1	Tbs. lemon juice	½	c. parsley, chopped fine

In small bowl, break up tomatoes with spoon. Add other salsa ingredients, cover and refrigerate to let flavors blend.

Sauté onions and green peppers in water or broth. Take the whole onion with cloves from beans and discard. Stir in sautéed onions and green peppers.

Serve over cooked rice. Top with salsa.

Unit 32: Salt

Chapter Summary

North Americans eat 10-20 times more salt than the body actually needs. High blood pressure, heart failure, and stroke are among the sad results. By avoiding highly salted foods and reeducating ourselves to enjoy meals with little or no salt, we take a giant step toward better health.

What Do You Have to Lose?

You can shed excess water, lower your blood pressure, protect yourself against stroke and heart disease—all this just by reducing the salt in your diet. It's a smart move. Are you ready to give it a try?

Cooking the Salt-free Way

It takes about three weeks for your tastes to adjust to a low-salt diet. During that time food can taste pretty bland. Stick with it, however, and you will be rewarded when the delicious, natural flavors of food come out of hiding.

Herbs Instead of Salt

Seasoning with herbs is an important skill for the health-conscious cook to master. Here are some suggestions to spice up your meals:

1. Use no more than ¼ teaspoon of dried herbs, or ¾ teaspoon of fresh herbs, for a dish that serves four people.

2. To soups and stews that are cooked a long time, add herbs during the last hour of cooking.

3. When cooking vegetables or making sauces and gravies, cook herbs along with them.

4. To cold foods such as tomato juice, salad dressings, and cottage cheese, add herbs several hours before serving. Storing these foods in the refrigerator for 3 to 4 hours deepens the flavor.

5. Remember that the correct combination of herbs and spices is the one that tastes best to you.

6. A very versatile seasoning is "Mrs. Dash." Use the one without salt and low in pepper.

7. Don't over season. Vegetables have wonderful flavors in their own right.

Seasoning Vegetables

Vegetables play a central role in the *Optimal Diet.* Here is a list of vegetables with some seasoning suggestions.

Seasonings for Vegetables

Asparagus: lemon juice, chives, thyme, tarragon.

Beans, dried: bay leaf, garlic, marjoram, onion, oregano.

Beans, green: basil, dill seed, thyme, onion, tarragon.

Beets: lemon juice or lemon peel.

Broccoli: lemon juice, dill, oregano.

Cabbage: creole cabbage with tomatoes, green pepper, garlic, and onion.

Carrots: parsley, mint, dillweed, lemon peel, sesame seed.

Cauliflower: Italian seasonings, paprika, sesame seed.

Celery: stir-fry with low-salt soy sauce, sesame seeds, and tomato.

Corn: bell pepper, pimiento, tomatoes, chives.

Okra: try broiling for a crisp texture.

Peas: fresh mushrooms, pearl onions, water chestnuts.

Potatoes: parsley, chopped green pepper, onion, chives.

Spinach: lemon juice, rosemary.

Squash: bake with chopped apple and lemon juice.

Tomatoes: sprinkle with curry powder; broil with mushrooms, green pepper, and onion.

This Week:

Use herbs instead of salt when you cook. Experiment with new seasonings for vegetables. The switch will increase the flavor of your food and decrease your risk of high blood pressure and stroke.

Unit 33: Vitamins and Minerals

Chapter Summary

The best place to get your vitamins is from fresh, whole foods. They're packed with the things your body needs for good health. Megadoses of vitamin supplements can be toxic. Don't upset your body's natural balance by taking too much of a good thing.

Nutritional Superstars

Do you know which 10 vegetables deliver the most vitamins and minerals per calorie? See if you can guess some of them. We will give you the answers at the end of this unit.

Health Doesn't Come in a Bottle

There is no potion or pill that can undo a lifetime of neglected health. Despite the claims of advertisers eager to make their fortune selling high-priced supplements, vitamin and mineral megadoses are not miracle cures.

Does This Make Sense?

People in western countries spend billions on processed and packaged foods which have many of their nutrients removed, and then turn around and pay fantastic prices for food supplements. Wouldn't it make more sense to eat the original, vitamin-packed foods instead?

You can't eat whole foods without getting a sizable dose of vitamins and minerals. A six-ounce potato, for example, contains 40 percent of the Recommended Daily Allowance of vitamin C, plus fiber, niacin, and potassium. It's a natural multi-vitamin.

Some Sources of Selected Nutrients

Nutrient	*Sources*
Vitamin A:	Dark-green and yellow vegetables; yellow fruit.
Vitamin B_1:	Whole grain products; peas; beans; wheat germ; potatoes; leafy vegetables.
Vitamin B_2:	Green leafy vegetables; whole grain products; prunes; milk (nonfat).
Vitamin B_3:	Whole grain and enriched breads and cereals; legumes; potatoes; green vegetables.
Vitamin B_{12}:	Dairy products (nonfat); enriched soy powder.
Vitamin C:	Cantaloupe, lemons, grapefruit, oranges, strawberries; raw cabbage, sweet peppers, tomatoes, potatoes.
Vitamin D:	Direct sunshine; fortified milk.
Vitamin E:	Whole grains; leafy vegetables; dairy products; sunflower seeds.
Iron:	Legumes; whole grain cereals and breads; dried fruits; green leafy vegetables.
Calcium & Phosphorus:	Greens: mustard, kale, turnip tops, cabbage, broccoli; whole grain products; citrus fruits; skim milk products.

Relax and Enjoy

All fresh fruits, whole grains, and vegetables provide an abundance of nutrients. If you eat a variety of these foods every day, your need for vitamins, minerals, and fiber is being met.

This Week:

Put a permanent check mark next to broccoli on your shopping list. One cup of this leafy green vegetable, cooked, has 165 percent of the RDA for vitamin C, 50 percent for vitamin A, 20 percent for calcium, plus iron, B vitamins, potassium, and other minerals.

Besides broccoli, other vegetables on the top 10 most nutritious list include peas, asparagus, cauliflower, sweet potatoes, carrots, corn, tomatoes, lettuce (except iceberg lettuce), and onions.

Unit 34: Stress

Chapter Summary

There are many things you can do to prevent stress from taking its toll. Regular exercise, a healthful diet, and stable life anchors, all play a part in combating the effects of physical and emotional pressure.

Overcoming Stress

Too much stress is a very real problem in our society. Learning to deal with it has become an important health issue since studies began linking stress to a host of physical ailments. In most cases, running away is not the answer. We must develop more positive methods of coping.

Chapter 34 of *Dynamic Living* lists seven ways to protect yourself against the harmful effects of stress. List the three suggestions that seem most valuable to you:

_____

_____

_____

What Can You Do?

Write two or three things you can do in the near future to put each of the suggestions you listed into action. Be specific. The more clearly you imagine an action or outcome, the easier it is to achieve it.

Suggestion 1

_____

_____

_____

_____

Suggestion 2

_____

_____

_____

_____

_____

Suggestion 3

_____

_____

_____

_____

_____

Handling Overload

Sometimes it is possible to feel emotionally stressed without knowing why. When that happens it is helpful to make a list of the things that are bothering you. Getting the sources of your stress onto paper allows you to focus and take action. Instead of overeating, overdrinking, or escaping into some time-wasting activity, you can identify the source of the problem and work toward a solution.

Stressed out because you have too many things on your "To Do" list? If so, start prioritizing your tasks. For each task on your list ask yourself if it is something that absolutely must be done. If it is, ask yourself if it must be done right now. Cutting your list down to its essentials will help get you through those times when life seems overwhelming.

This Week:

In this unit you listed specific actions that can help you cope with the stressful world we live in. This week, get them off the page and working for you.

Unit 35: Depression

Chapter Summary

Improving physical health, pursuing worthwhile goals, developing positive mental attitudes and spiritual values can help people deal with their feelings of depression and hopelessness.

Strategies for Beating the Blues

Chapter 35 of *Dynamic Living* presents some strategies for beating the blues. List those that might be useful to you in the spaces below.

_____

_____

_____

_____

The Power to Choose

One of the things that sets us apart from other creatures is our ability to make choices. We do not simply respond by instinct when faced with a situation. We can think about our actions and choose between alternatives.

You have been exercising this birthright while working through the practical exercises in this book. By choosing to eat foods that prevent disease, by exercising, by your willingness to learn, you are making choices that can improve your health and energy.

Everyday Choices

Your health is not the only area where wise choices return big dividends. The decisions you make in other areas of your life are equally important for maintaining a positive outlook.

A Higher Power

Through the ages, millions have found comfort in time of need by turning to a Higher Power for strength and wisdom. Stories of people overcoming problems that seemed unsolvable are abundant. Alcoholics Anonymous and other recovery programs recognize this and have included acceptance of the Higher Power concept as an important part of their programs. They recognize this power as a source of meaning, hope, and inspiration that cannot be taken away by circumstance.

It is easy for the hustle and bustle of life to crowd out time for spiritual nourishment. Yet those who have endured trying times can vouch for these values. Is your spiritual life the source of inspiration, strength, and renewal that it could be?

Family and Social Relationships

We humans are social creatures. We need the sense of community and belonging that comes from our relationship to others. When we feel isolated or in conflict it is much easier to slip into depression.

Think of the important relationships in your life. Imagine that each of them represents a bank account—an emotional bank account. Acts of love, kindness, understanding, and respect are deposits to these accounts; acts of selfishness, impatience, anger, and neglect are withdrawals.

Now think of a specific relationship. What could you do this week to add to its emotional bank account?

_____

_____

This Week:

Make some deposits in the emotional bank accounts of those close to you. Use the ideas you listed to invest in happy, satisfying relationships.

Unit 36: Emotions

Chapter Summary

The body makes its own "feel good" substances, endorphins, that are both protective and health promoting. Physical exercise and a positive mental attitude boost the production of these endorphins in the brain and increase the body's ability to fight disease.

The Happiness Quiz
Part 1

It's easier to be happy when you feel healthy. Which of the following are you doing to physically boost your state of mind?

❑ *Exercise daily:* (preferably in the fresh air) Studies show that exercise is one of the most effective cures for the blues. Certainly, it is the least expensive.

❑ *Avoid caffeine:* Too much caffeine shortens your fuse and decreases your tolerance to life's stresses. It can also cause insomnia, robbing your body of much needed rest.

❑ *Avoid alcohol:* Alcohol is a depressant, yet many people turn to it during periods when they are experiencing negative emotions. That is a little like throwing gasoline on a fire. You don't need a depressant when you are feeling down.

❑ *Eat a low-fat diet:* Build it around whole grains, vegetables, and fruits. On this diet you will feel better, look better, and have more energy. All of these benefits create an environment where positive emotions can flourish.

❑ *Get enough fresh air:* A well-ventilated house and frequent deep breathing helps keep your blood oxygenated. This is essential for being mentally and emotionally in top form. Fresh supplies of oxygen help keep you awake and alert.

Part 2

The mind and body are linked. Just as it is difficult to be happy when you are feeling the effects of physical illness, it's also hard to feel healthy when you are in conflict with yourself or others.

The following habits cultivate a happy, thankful attitude. How many of them are you developing?

❏ *Count your blessings:* Every one of us has much to be thankful for. Paying attention to what is good in your life rather than being overwhelmed by troubles is one key to a joyful existence.

❏ *Work toward harmony in relationships:* If you nurture the negative emotions of bitterness, envy, and jealousy toward others, you rob yourself of much joy. On the other hand, developing a forgiving, caring attitude brings happiness and friendship into your life.

❏ *Work for the good of others:* Reaching out beyond yourself to touch others helps you as much as it does those whose lives you brighten. Your emotional focus moves away from your own problems and you feel good about yourself.

❏ *Take time for spiritual renewal:* The great men and women of all times have drawn strength and inspiration from their faith in something greater than themselves. This faith has helped them overcome obstacles and achieve greatness. Pausing from the rush of everyday life to contemplate the deeper things, reaching out to a power beyond one's self may be the most effective means of bringing happiness back into one's life.

This Week:

Look back over the Happiness Quiz. Are there things that you aren't doing that might give your emotional life a boost? Choose one item and focus on it this week.

Unit 37: Mind Power

Chapter Summary

Thoughts and emotions directly influence the mind, which in turn, affects the body. Research suggests that a stable emotional life is as important to good health as more traditional factors such as exercise and diet.

Questions Are the Answer

We've seen that the mind and emotions have a powerful influence in our physical lives. But how do we harness that power to work for us? One answer is through the power of questions.

Questions Have the Power to Focus

A question is like a lens, turning the focus of your attention toward a specific problem or situation. When you ask yourself a question, your mind automatically goes to work looking for an answer.

The right questions can affect all areas of your life—from your relationships, to your attitudes, to your creativity and ability to solve problems.

Five Powerful Questions

Here are five questions that only you can answer. If you back your answers up with action, each of them can have a tremendous effect on your life. Be specific, and ask yourself the following:

1. What is the one thing I could do that would have the greatest positive, long-term effect on my life?

_____

_____

_____

2. What is one thing I could do that would improve my relationship with someone I care about?

_____

_____

_____

3. Ask this one often: What is there in my life, right now, that is worth being happy about?

_____

_____

_____

4. What can I do today to develop a more healthful lifestyle?

_____

_____

_____

5. Here's one to ask yourself when you are in a bind: If it were someone else in my situation, what would I tell them to do?

Don't Ask Yourself Negative Questions

Don't ask yourself questions like, "Why am I so dumb?" Or "Why can't I stick to an exercise program?" Those questions focus your mind in a negative direction. Instead, rephrase them in a positive, productive way: "What can I do in the future to avoid this mistake?" Or "How can I adjust my schedule to make exercising easier?"

This Week:

Use the five questions listed in this chapter and try to come up with several more of your own. You will be surprised at the power of this simple technique.

Unit 38: Plant Food

Chapter Summary

Vegetarians are no longer viewed as food fanatics and counter-culture oddballs. Studies confirm that most live longer, healthier lives, and that their diets are more ecologically sound. Making the transition to a meat-free diet can be a challenging adventure, leading to a new level of good health and well being.

The *Optimal Diet*

By now you have been exposed to the *Optimal Diet* several times. Are you applying the guidelines for good health listed in the summary of *Dynamic Living?* Here are some questions to see how much you remember:

1. Animal products are necessary for good health and nutrition.

    __ True
    __ False

2. The average risk of heart disease for a man eating meat, eggs, and dairy products is

    __ 15%
    __ 35%
    __ 50%
    __ 75%

3. On average, vegetarians are

    __ Heavier than meat eaters
    __ Thinner than meat eaters
    __ Weigh the same as meat eaters

4. Most of the calories in meat come from

    __ Fat
    __ Protein
    __ Carbohydrates

5. Cholesterol is found in

__ All foods
__ Peanut butter
__ All animal products
__ Foods that come from plant sources

6. A diet high in flesh foods has been linked with

__ Heart disease
__ Stroke
__ Cancer
__ All of the above

Lunch on the Go

For busy people, lunch is often a difficult meal. The temptation is to grab something quick. Fortunately, quick does not have to mean a burger from a fast-food restaurant. With some advance planning, you can take a healthful lunch wherever you go. Here are tips for taking the *Optimal Diet* on the road.

Bring a thermos: A thermos lets you carry along delicious soups and stews. Who said lunch had to be built around a sandwich?

Resealable plastic containers: Tupperware-type containers are excellent for raw, cut vegetables, salads, and leftovers. Be creative!

Microwave it: If you have access to a microwave, bring a potato and some type of topping for lunch. It takes just minutes for a nutritious, piping hot meal. Who knows, your example could inspire a lunchtime trend toward good eating.

This Week:

Meat can be hazardous to your health. Start eliminating it from your diet by making your own delicious lunches.

Answers

1. False   2. 50%   3. Thinner   4. Fat   5. Animal products
6. All of above

Unit 39: Digestion

Chapter Summary

Digestion is a marvelous process. To help your body work with maximum efficiency, space meals four to five hours apart and avoid snacking.

No More Rolaids

How do you spell relief? If you are like most North Americans you spell it D-O-L-L-A-R-S. Each year we spend millions on pills and potions to quiet our angry stomachs. There is a better way, of course—stop overloading your stomach and give it the rest it needs.

Sweetening a Sour Stomach

How often does your stomach protest?

__ Never
__ Several times a year
__ Several times a month
__ Weekly
__ Every day

If you frequently have indigestion or an upset stomach, and your doctor has ruled out more serious problems, it may be your eating habits that are causing you grief.

Answer the following questions with a yes or no.

1. ___ Do you have regular eating times?

Your body thrives on a regular schedule, not only of eating, but of waking, sleeping, and exercise.

2. ___ Do you often eat between meals?

When new food shows up in a stomach that is already working, digestion must slow down until the system deals with the new arrival.

Imagine a washing machine working on a load of clothes. If you come by every 10 minutes, turn the dial back, and dump in more clothes, you would never finish a load. A washing machine, just like your stomach, needs time to finish its cycle.

3. __ Are your meals spaced 4-5 hours apart?

Spacing meals several hours apart allows the stomach to work at its own pace. Food from one meal is completely digested before the next one arrives.

4. __ Do you drink coffee?

Coffee, even decaf, contains substances that can irritate the lining of the stomach. Too much of this substance can send your stomach into rebellion.

5. __ Do you eat right before going to bed?

The stomach, like the rest of your body, needs rest. A meal or snack late in the evening forces it to work overtime.

Dealing With Gas

Many people adjusting to a high-fiber diet experience problems with intestinal gas. This is especially true when legumes are on the menu. Here are some suggestions that can help:

For occasional intestinal gas, try some pharmaceutical-grade charcoal. It adsorbs gas and provides a measure of relief. It is available as powder, tablets, syrup, or capsules and is sold over the counter.

To reduce gas caused by cooked dried beans, try soaking them overnight, discarding the soak water, and replacing it with fresh water for cooking.

This Week:

Give your stomach a break by spacing meals further apart. Not interrupting the digestive cycle with snacks will sweeten the disposition of a cranky stomach.

Unit 40: Fighting Fads

Chapter Summary

Preoccupation with new discoveries and "quick fixes" focuses attention away from the need for a healthy lifestyle and well-balanced diet. There is no single food that will cure a lifetime of poor health choices. Only by adopting a balanced lifestyle can one begin to enjoy the many benefits of good health.

Slanting the News

Oat bran is an example of what can happen when the media or food companies blow a study out of proportion. Often they do it without regard for the significance or reliability of the findings.

Bread Packaging

Food companies are experts at manipulating the truth. They don't necessarily lie, but they often do slant the truth in their favor by publicizing only that which supports their purposes.

Imagine that you design packaging for a large bread company. Your instructions are to create a new wrapper for the company's loaves of white bread. When shoppers see the wrapper, you want them to choose your bread over that of the competition. What kinds of things could you put on the wrapper to convince people to buy your bread?

Your market research shows that consumers associate the words "whole wheat" with good nutrition. The bread you are selling isn't made from whole-wheat flour, but your research also shows that many customers think the words "whole wheat" and "100% wheat" mean the same thing. They don't. "Whole wheat" means the flour used came from the whole wheat grain, while "100% wheat" means only that the flour used came from wheat rather than some other grain.

You put the words "100% Wheat Bread" in large letters on the wrapper and it works. More customers buy your loaf of bread, feeling confident that they are choosing a nutritious loaf. You win, but at your customer's expense.

How Do You Decide?

With so many people slanting the health news for their own purposes, how do we know what to believe? Good common sense is one answer. When you read about the results of a study or hear the claims of an advertiser, ask yourself the following questions:

Believability Checklist

1. Who is making this claim? Be suspicious if it is the producer of the product.

2. What do they have to gain by publicizing this information? What is their motive?

3. Do other studies agree with these claims or is this an exception or "new" finding being picked up by the media? The news media loves a sensational story. As a result, they often publish the results of flawed or biased studies.

4. Does the claim sound like magic? If it sounds too good to be true, chances are it is.

5. Is a drug or food touted as reversing a chronic condition brought on by long-term lifestyle patterns? Beware of the quick fix.

6. Does the claim contradict the principles of balance and common sense?

This Week:

Look at health news with a critical eye. Use the Believability Checklist to screen out misinformation.

Unit 41: Breakfast

Chapter Summary

A good breakfast boosts your energy, increases your attention span, and heightens your sense of well-being. Recent studies have even linked healthy breakfasts with less chronic disease, increased longevity, and better health.

Make the Most of Your Day

Many studies have emphasized the importance of breakfast. If you want to make the most of your day, fuel your body with the right stuff. The following questions will help you examine your morning eating habits.

The Breakfast Quiz

1. Do you skip breakfast often? Mom was right—breakfast really is the most important meal of the day. If you skip it, you are starting the day at a disadvantage.

2. Do you get up in time to eat a good breakfast? If not, how could you change your routine to give yourself time for a nutritious morning meal?

   _____

   _____

3. Are you hungry in the morning or is your appetite a late riser? Chapter 41 of *Dynamic Living* offers two solutions to this problem. What are they?

   _____

   _____

4. Is your usual breakfast high in fiber from whole fruits and grains? The fiber and complex carbohydrates in whole foods provides a steady release of energy that most processed breakfast foods lack. It will keep you going strong all morning.

5. Is your breakfast high in fats and cholesterol? A traditional breakfast of eggs and sausage can be the most deadly meal of the day. Breakfast meats are loaded with fats, cholesterol, and salt. Eggs can send your cholesterol skyrocketing. The sausage and egg breakfast needs to go the way of the dinosaur if you want to avoid extinction.

How Well Have You Been Eating?

What did you have for breakfast this morning? In the spaces below, list everything you ate.

_____

_____

_____

Based on what you have learned, how can you improve the quality of your breakfasts?

_____

_____

_____

This Week:

Make eating a good breakfast a priority. Note any changes in your energy level and productivity. The recipe below will help get you started.

Cashew Oat Waffles

Blenderize the following ingredients until smooth. Bake in a preheated waffle iron for 10-12 minutes:

2 c. water	1½ c. regular rolled oats
⅓ c. raw cashews	½ t. salt

Top with mashed bananas, fresh or frozen berries, apple sauce, or crushed pineapple.

Unit 42: Exercise

Chapter Summary

Exercise slows down the aging process. It strengthens the heart, lowers blood pressure, relieves stress, and helps you maintain a desirable weight. You don't need expensive equipment or a health club membership to start. Walking can provide all these benefits and more.

How Do You Rate?

How would you rate your level of fitness?

__ High: I have a regular exercise program.

__ Medium: Sometimes exercise, but not regularly.

__ Low: I don't exercise; I rest.

The 10-Step Exercise Program

Have you tried exercise before and found that you just couldn't stick with it? If so, you should try the world's easiest exercise system. It's called the 10-Step Program.

All you do is make a commitment to the first 10 steps of a daily walk. That's it. You get out and take those steps every day. Once they're behind you, you can turn around and go home, if you wish.

The system works because it eases you past those difficult first steps. It gets you up and going, and if you are like most people, once you get going you will finish the entire walk.

Another reason the 10-Step Program is valuable is that it keeps you in the habit of exercising even when you can't manage your full routine. You might be sick, or traveling, yet in almost every situation you can manage 10 steps. In this way you maintain the exercise habit even when you can't exercise. That's important if you want to enjoy the benefits of fitness for the rest of your life.

Plan Ahead

Another useful technique is to plan your exercise sessions in advance. Make an appointment with yourself for at least 30 minutes—longer if you are exercising to lose weight. If you are an early riser try exercising before breakfast. If your morning is already too full, walk during your lunch hour or in the evening. The important thing is to find a time that is right for you.

People Make Exercise Fun

Many people complain that exercise is boring. To liven up your sessions, include friends and family members in your exercise activities. If they won't join you, take the dog out for a stroll. Exercise can be enjoyable if you approach it with an attitude of fun and creativity.

This Week:

Schedule your exercise sessions in advance and use the 10-Step Program to get you moving. Regular exercise is as necessary as air, water, and wholesome food. Don't let another week go by without it.

Unit 43: Super Fluid

Chapter Summary

Today, North Americans drink more soft drinks and alcoholic beverages than water. These substitutes force the body to deal with calories and chemicals, and can disturb the process of digestion. The body needs water to function properly. When you want refreshment, choose the real thing—water.

Eight Is Too Much

Sandy had made up her mind. She was going to give her body the water it needed: eight glasses a day, without fail. Opening the cupboard she selected a large tumbler. This, she decided, would be her glass.

Things didn't go well for Sandy that day. Eight glasses turned out to be a lot of water. When she wasn't sipping, she was scurrying down the hall to the bathroom.

No wonder people don't drink enough water, thought Sandy. *I feel like a sponge.*

Size Makes a Difference

Sandy was making things difficult for herself. If she had taken time to measure she would have found that the glass she had selected held 16 ounces of liquid—two cups of water. Instead of drinking the eight, 8-ounce glasses recommended, she was drinking twice that amount.

Sandy switched to a smaller cup. Now she gets the water she needs without wearing a path to the bathroom.

Most People Should Drink More

Water really is the most healthful drink. We can live only a few days without it. Even though we all get enough to sustain us, most people don't drink enough for optimum functioning. We sip enough to survive, when we should be drinking enough to thrive. The result is unnecessary stress placed on the body's cleansing system and other functions.

Are You Convinced?

After reading chapter 43 in *Dynamic Living,* do you feel that drinking more water is something you need to do?

Start Early

One way to make sure you get your daily quota is by drinking two glasses of water when you wake up in the morning. Do this before you get caught up in the activities of the day. With two glasses down, you only need to drink four to six more during the rest of the day. That is a feat everyone can manage.

Fill Up Often

Are there other times in the day when it would be convenient for you to take a water break? If you wait until you are thirsty, you probably won't get enough.

In the spaces below, list times when it would be convenient for you to stop and have a drink. Once you make these pauses a habit, your body will always have the fluid it needs.

_____

_____

_____

_____

This Week:

Drink six to eight glasses of water each day this week, but make sure the glasses are the right size. An 8-ounce glass (1 cup) is recommended. Be good to yourself: start enjoying nature's super fluid today.

Unit 44: Bottled or Tap?

Chapter Summary

In most cases, the health hazards we face from not drinking enough water are greater than those from possible contaminants in the water supply. If you are concerned, have your water tested, or install a good charcoal filter. A filter helps purify your water and makes it taste better.

Danger From the Sky

The family was gathered around the television for the evening when it happened. A violent explosion ripped a hole through the ceiling and something heavy crashed to the floor beside them. What could have caused this unexpected intrusion?

The source, as it turned out, was a commercial jet with leaky plumbing. While the plane was at high altitude, liquid had seeped out and frozen on the side of the plane. As the plane descended, the ice thawed and came loose. The result was a deadly sewage bomb, and a narrow miss.

Hazards, Hazards, Everywhere

Do you ever get the feeling that you are at risk? Hardly a day goes by without some report announcing a new danger to worry about. It seems that just about everything we eat, drink, breathe, or touch is hazardous to our health. It can be overwhelming—not to mention confusing.

What are some of the health hazards you have heard about lately?

_____

_____

_____

_____

Can You Know Too Much?

Is there a danger in being aware of so many potential hazards? Perhaps. Some people say, "Everything is harmful. Why make it worse by worrying?"

Fighting Where the Battle Is

While it's true that we can't protect ourselves from every conceivable danger, there is much we can do. Heart disease strikes every other person in the United States. Cancer and diabetes afflict millions more. Lack of exercise makes most of us old before our time. It is with these dangers that we should concern ourselves most.

What makes more sense, reinforcing your roof against the one-in-a-billion chance that a passing airplane may drop a frozen sewage bomb, or starting a regular exercise program?

What makes more sense, eating fruits and vegetables needed for good health, or avoiding them on the off chance that they may contain pesticide residue?

What makes more sense, drinking the eight glasses of water that your body needs to flush out toxins, or avoiding tap water for fear that it may contain something dangerous?

Good Insurance

A healthy body provides good insurance against the dangers that we may face. The body's ability to heal and protect itself is truly remarkable.

This Week:

Before you let a headline panic you, make sure you know how serious a threat is involved. Take action if warranted; otherwise, relax in the knowledge that your new lifestyle is boosting your body's ability to protect itself.

Unit 45: Sunlight

Chapter Summary

Sunshine can be good for you. It kills germs, helps improve your mood, and allows the body to produce vitamin D. Yet, while some exposure is good, too much can destroy the skin's elasticity and increase the risk of skin cancer. Enjoy sunlight and outside activities, but protect yourself from overexposure.

Friend or Foe?

Over the last few years, articles about the effects of the sun and the danger of skin cancer have driven many people into the dark. That's not all bad. Certainly you should use caution to avoid burning, but to avoid the sun altogether deprives you of one of nature's great healing remedies.

Ask Yourself

How often do you spend time in the sunshine?

__ Every day, weather permitting

__ Most days

__ A few times a week

__ Rarely

It's good to spend at least a few minutes in the sunshine every day. Studies have shown that, for some people, lack of exposure to light causes depression. For everyone, taking a sunshine break gives your body a dose of vitamin D and acts as a disinfectant, killing bacteria on your clothes and skin.

During the summer do you:

__ Sizzle and sunburn?

__ Work on a deep, dark tan?

__ Tan lightly?

__ Stay out of the sun completely?

If you sizzle and burn or go for that deep tan, watch out! You are putting yourself at risk for skin cancer and damaging the elasticity of your skin.

On the other hand, lightly tanned skin is more resistant to sunburn and less prone to infection. Get outside in the fresh air. Soak up a little sunshine each day; just don't overdo it.

When it is bright outside, do you open up your curtains and let the sun into your home?

___ Always

___ Sometimes

___ Never

Open up your windows and let the sunshine in. It will kill germs, lift your spirits, and enhance your health.

Sunlight Suggestions

1. Avoid going to sleep in the sun. It's a recipe for a severe sunburn.

2. Use sunscreen and sunglasses to protect yourself. A hat is also helpful to shade your face when you are working outdoors.

3. Be extra careful when you are around water or on snow. The reflection from these surfaces can increase your exposure, causing you to burn rapidly.

4. If you are swimming, remember to reapply your sunscreen when you are finished. Better yet, use waterproof sunscreen.

This Week:

Get some sunshine every day. Combined with exercise in the fresh air, sunlight is one of nature's most effective remedies.

Unit 46: Tobacco

Chapter Summary

Tobacco is the deadliest drug in the world. In the United States alone it kills over 400,000 people a year. Eighty percent of lung cancers could be prevented if people stopped smoking. The biggest favor people can do for themselves is to break the smoking habit.

Kicking the Habit

The first step in breaking any habit is to decide that you are going to change. It's not enough just to want to change or to imagine that you will change someday. Breaking an addiction to tobacco requires positive commitment.

Weigh the Evidence

When making a life-changing decision, it helps to look at the pros and cons of the situation. There actually are some reasons to continue smoking.

Reasons to Keep Using Tobacco

1. Tobacco gives a pleasurable sensation of soothing relaxation and well-being.

2. Tobacco suppresses the appetite, making it easier to keep excess weight off.

3. Quitting can be a disruptive, uncomfortable, and stressful process.

4. Lighting up is a good excuse to take a break.

5. Trying to quit, and failing, hurts the smoker's self-esteem.

These are some pretty powerful reasons to keep smoking, especially when combined with physical and psychological addiction to nicotine. Anyone who faces these issues and overcomes them deserves respect and admiration.

Reasons to Quit Smoking

While there are some reasons to keep smoking, there are far more persuasive reasons to stop— reasons that convince thousands to quit each year. Here are just a few:

1. Quitting is the single most important thing you can do for your health and longevity.

2. Reduced risk of heart disease, stroke, and cancer of the lungs, mouth, throat, pancreas, bladder, kidneys, and cervix.

3. Reduced risk of emphysema and osteoporosis.

4. Elimination of the risk posed to the smoker's family from second-hand smoke.

5. Less chance of a smoker's children and grandchildren smoking.

6. Better breath, whiter teeth, and fewer wrinkles.

7. Less time spent sick; more physical endurance.

8. Lower medical and insurance costs.

The list goes on, and it grows every year as we learn more about the harmful effects of tobacco.

To Smoke or Not to Smoke

If you smoke, what will it take for you to quit? If you don't smoke, what was it that kept you from starting or helped you give it up?

_____

_____

_____

_____

This Week:

If you smoke, get information about the different methods of breaking the habit. Choose your method, set your goal, then do it! Some can quit cold turkey, others get help in a stop-smoking program.

Unit 47: Alcohol

Chapter Summary

Alcohol extracts a heavy price from personal health. This goes for teens as well as adults. Young people who grow up in nonalcoholic homes are less likely to have problems with alcohol when they reach adulthood. A parent's example can make a big difference.

The World's Most Abused Drug

Alcohol is not just a problem for young people; it's the greatest drug problem in the world for all ages. In the United States it's second only to tobacco on the list of most deadly drugs.

Despite the dangers, everyone in our society comes into contact with alcoholic beverages. If nothing else, we are exposed to commercials on television singing the praises of one brew after another.

Getting a Clear Picture

If you drink, it can be helpful to review your drinking habits periodically. The following questions are designed to bring them into focus.

1. In what situations do you use alcohol?

   __ Never, I don't drink
   __ To unwind after work
   __ At social gatherings
   __ On special occasions: birthdays, anniversaries
   __ With meals at restaurants
   __ At taverns or bars

2. How often do you drink alcohol?

   __ A few times a year
   __ A few times a month
   __ Several times a week
   __ On weekends
   __ Every day

3. When you drink, how much do you consume at one sitting?

　　__ 1 drink

　　__ 2 drinks

　　__ 3 or 4 drinks

　　__ 5 or more

Are You Satisfied?

How satisfied are you with your answers? Do they represent the behaviors you value? If not, what could you change?

_____

_____

_____

Alcohol and Nutrition

Throughout this workbook we have urged you to avoid highly refined products that are high in calories but low in nutrition. Alcohol certainly falls into this category. Two cans of beer, for example, carry 300 calories; two jiggers of 100 proof whiskey, 250 calories; two glasses of dessert wine pack 280 calories—and they are all empty calories, providing none of the nutrients your body requires.

Altogether, alcohol accounts for 9 percent of the calories in the American diet. No wonder we are overfed and undernourished.

This Week:

Make this "ban the booze" week at your house. You should be able to get through it without any sort of urge or discomfort.

If you can't, you need to seriously consider who is the master: you or the alcohol. If you can get through the week with no problems, why not quit altogether? It will help keep your weight under control, improve your nutrition, and set a good example for the young people in your life.

Unit 48: Caffeine

Chapter Summary

Caffeine is an addictive drug. It produces physical and mental effects when withdrawn. While an occasional small dose of caffeine may not make a difference, heavier use has been linked to health problems.

Coffee: Food or Drug?

Imagine going to buy coffee at the grocery store and finding the coffee section missing.

"What's going on?" you ask the clerk. "Where is the coffee?"

"Oh, haven't you heard? Coffee has been classified as a drug. The pharmacist sells it now."

Shaking your head in disbelief, you walk across the store to where the pharmacist dispenses medications, drugs, and—caffeinated beverages.

The pharmacist smiles at you knowingly. "You look like you're here for some coffee. I can tell from your expression."

You nod and tell him what brand you would like.

"That's fine," he says. "No prescription necessary—I just need to type up the warning label."

"Warning label?"

"That's right. Just the usual. It says—

Warning: This drink contains caffeine. Possible side effects include addiction, tremors, nervousness, anxiety, insomnia, chronic fatigue, lack of energy, stomach irritation, vomiting, interference with calcium and iron absorption, and the aggravation of ulcers."

He hands you the coffee, but you decline. "No thanks," you say. "I think I've changed my mind."

Are You an Addict?

You could be a caffeine addict without even knowing it. Here are some questions and a suggestion to help you find out.

Do you frequently consume any of the following?

__ Coffee

__ Tea

__ Chocolate

__ Caffeinated soft drinks

How important is a cup of coffee in the morning?

__ Essential: can't get going without it.

__ Important: helps jump-start the day.

__ Enjoyable: it's pleasant once in a while.

__ What's coffee? I never touch the stuff.

One way to find out if you are addicted is to stop all caffeine intake for a week. If you're hooked, chances are good that you will notice physical symptoms like headache, lack of appetite, and nausea, which can last from one to five days. Psychologically, you may feel down and listless, and of course, there will be a strong urge for your favorite beverage.

Breaking the Habit

If you find you're a caffeine fiend, here are a few things you can do to ease through withdrawal.

1. Drink plenty of fresh water.

2. Slow down your daily activities.

3. Exercise in the fresh air.

4. Get the support of others around you.

5. Reward yourself for taking such a positive step.

This Week:

Skip the caffeinated drinks like tea, coffee, and cola. See how you fare. At the end of the week review this material and give serious consideration to making your body a caffeine-free zone.

Unit 49: Drugs

Chapter Summary

Many people have a childlike faith in drugs and medicines. They take them for every conceivable ailment. But using big-gun medicines for flyswatter problems, or for problems that should be solved by lifestyle measures, can leave you tired, depleted, and depressed. Use drugs sparingly and with care.

Pain Is a Warning

Too many people run to the medicine cabinet whenever they feel the slightest ache or pain. They don't realize that pain often acts as a warning system, telling us something is wrong.

We may be eating too much, drinking too much, smoking too much, or taking on obligations beyond our capacities. When pain is blocked by drugs, we ignore these causes rather than changing the behaviors that cause the pain in the first place. This kind of neglect sets the stage for more serious diseases.

Two Categories of Drugs

In chapter 49, *Dynamic Living* divides drugs into two categories: those that attack the cause of the problem, and those that help relieve symptoms.

If you take any medications, list them in the spaces below. Write a "C" next to those that attack the cause of the problem. Put an "S" by those that simply help relieve symptoms.

_____

_____

_____

_____

_____

The Drug Checklist

Before you take any drug, there are a few things you should find out:

1. Is the drug absolutely necessary?

2. Will the drug conflict with other medications you are already taking?

3. Exactly how long will you need to take the drug?

4. What are the possible risks and side effects associated with the drug? (No medication is completely safe. Even aspirin can have side effects.)

5. Is there a nondrug alternative? (Many problems can be controlled by lifestyle measures.)

6. Is addiction possible with this drug? (Drugs prescribed for pain, anxiety, or sleep disorders are habit forming.)

When Drugs Are Necessary

When you need to take a drug, here are some things to keep in mind.

1. Don't quit taking it unless you get approval from your physician. Many drugs need to be taken for a certain period of time. Quitting early can render the treatment ineffective.

2. Don't take a larger dosage than you are prescribed. It's not true that if a little of something is good, more is better. In fact, more can be deadly. Take your medications only as directed.

3. Let your doctor know that you would prefer not to take drugs if possible.

This Week:

Don't go running to the medicine cabinet for every little ache and pain. The cure is often worse than the problem. When you must take a drug, be sure you get the answers to the questions on the drug checklist.

Dynamic Living

Unit 50: Air

Chapter Summary

The human body operates on oxygen. Make sure yours gets enough by exercising, keeping your house well ventilated, and pausing frequently to take slow, deep breaths.

Air Inventory

Right now, without changing anything about the way you are sitting or breathing, answer the following questions:

1. How are you sitting right now? Is your spine straight, or are you slouching? Are your shoulders rolled forward?

2. Observe your breathing for a few moments. Is it shallow or deep?

3. Do the clothes you are wearing, or the chair you are sitting in, restrict your breathing?

4. Is the room you are in well ventilated with fresh air, or is it closed and stuffy?

5. Is there cigarette smoke or heavy smog in the air?

6. Have you (or will you) exercise today?

7. Have you eaten a high-fat meal today? (A high-fat meal reduces your blood's ability to carry oxygen.)

8. When was the last time you got up and moved around? Have you taken a break or done some deep breathing during the last couple hours?

Running on Oxygen

Oxygen is vital to each of the trillions of cells that make up your body. Poor breathing habits, or poor air to breathe, can rob the body of this vital element. Bad air and poor breathing habits promote negative emotions like depression and irritability. It can also cause headaches and chronic feelings of fatigue and exhaustion.

Breathe Deeply

Take a moment to try this simple breathing exercise. It will energize and refresh you.

Stand or sit with your back straight. Exhale deeply through your mouth. Now, draw the air back into your lungs. As you do, imagine it going right down into your belly, filling it. Feel your stomach expand as you inhale.

When your lungs are full, slowly begin to exhale. Tighten the muscles of your stomach as you gently push the last bit of air out.

Repeat the process, slowly, five or six times.

Do this exercise when you wake in the morning and several times during the day. If possible, step outdoors into the fresh air. Refresh body and mind by giving yourself a caffeine-free boost.

This Week:

Practice breathing deep, and experiment with the other tips listed in chapter 50 of *Dynamic Living*.

Unit 51: Rest

Chapter Summary

Rest is an important part of life's rhythm. Most adults do best with seven to eight hours of sleep each night. If you have trouble sleeping, don't reach for sleep medications. Take a warm, relaxing bath. Exercise daily. Maintain a regular schedule. Strive for a clear conscience and tranquil mind.

Sleep Quiz

Feeling tired? Have a hard time getting out of bed in the morning? The following questions are designed to get you thinking about your sleep habits.

1. I have trouble falling asleep at night.

    a. Usually
    b. Often
    c. Rarely
    d. Never

2. I usually get enough sleep and awake feeling rested.

    a. Usually
    b. Often
    c. Rarely
    d. Never

3. I use caffeinated drinks (like coffee and soft drinks).

    a. More than 10 cups/day
    b. 5-9 cups/day
    c. 2-4 cups/day
    d. Less than 2 cups/day

4. I go to bed at night early enough to get a good night's sleep.

    a. Always
    b. Often
    c. Rarely
    d. Never

Trouble Falling Asleep

Many people occasionally have trouble falling asleep. Three common reasons for this are emotional stress, caffeine, and lack of exercise. Fortunately, all of these can be controlled.

Caffeine, found in coffee, tea, and many soft drinks can be reduced or eliminated from the diet.

Emotional stress can also be reduced by handling disturbing problems earlier in the day, when you are rested. Don't wait till bedtime to bring up problems.

A regular exercise program may be the best medicine of all for ensuring a good night's rest. It reduces stress and provides a pleasant physical fatigue that helps you sleep soundly.

Getting Enough Sleep

For many, getting to sleep isn't the problem—making time for it is. Busy schedules, bolstered by strong coffee, cut into the hours needed for sleep.

Your body is your most valuable possession. It may be tempting to skip sleep, but in the long run that is counter productive. A parable by Stephen Covey from his book *The Seven Habits of Highly Effective People* illustrates this point:

Imagine you are walking through the woods and you come upon a man feverishly trying to saw down a tree. The man looks exhausted. He says he has been sawing on the same tree for five hours.

"Why don't you take a break for a couple minutes and sharpen that saw?" you ask. "It will cut faster."

"No time for that," he gasps. "I'm too busy sawing."

This Week:

Sharpen your saw by allowing yourself enough time to rest. Set a regular time to wake up, and go to bed early enough to get seven or eight hours of sleep. If you do, you'll find that you are able to accomplish more during your waking hours.

Unit 52: Trust in Divine Power

Chapter Summary

The ultimate lifestyle includes not just health and fitness, but spiritual growth. Trust in God supplies a missing piece in our lives. It brings quality, fulfillment, and hope for the future.

Beyond Good Health

Throughout this workbook we have presented ideas that can have a profound effect on your physical life. But good health is not the pinnacle of existence. Many who are otherwise healthy carry within them a deep longing for something more. At the root of our being is the need for greater purpose and meaning in life.

The Spiritual Dimension

Where do you turn for renewal? What is at your core, your center of being? The testimony of our history is clear: those who were most content in life drew strength and renewal from a source larger than themselves. They perceived the touch of the infinite in the beauty of nature, the wisdom of a holy book, or in the private stillness of meditation and prayer.

The spiritual dimension of life is an area about which science has little to say. Yet poets, wise men, and our own hearts affirm its importance.

Time

Like all things of value, cultivating the spiritual side of our nature takes an investment of time. Attention must be shifted from immediate concerns to deeper, more eternal issues. We need to take time for stillness, away from the commotion and noise of our everyday lives.

We need time to explore the deeper side of ourselves, to read inspiring words, or just to walk in the sunshine and fresh air.

When was the last time you allowed yourself to really enjoy the people closest to you? How long has it been since you joined with others who find faith and inspiration in a Higher Power?

Spiritual Growth

What are some things you could do to enhance your spiritual life?

_____

_____

_____

_____

_____

_____

_____

This Week:

This week take some time to step back and think about what is truly important to you. Look beyond the clamor of daily activity to the universal themes of life. Choose an inspiring book, listen to some uplifting music, give thanks for the marvelous gift of life and health. Every breath you take is a miracle. Every morning is a new start.

Testing Your Knowledge

1. Every cigarette smoked shortens a smoker's life by ___ minutes.
   a. 3   b. 6   c. 12   d. 20

2. In the last 15 years, the number of super-fat children has _____.
   a. decreased   b. increased slightly   c. doubled   d. tripled

3. The western diet contains about _____ of cholesterol/day.
   a. 100 mg   b. 300 mg   c. 500 mg   d. 800 mg

4. An obese man is _____ times more likely to have a heart attack by age 60 than a man of normal weight.
   a. 1.5   b. 3   c. 5

5. By definition, obese means being _____ or more above ideal weight.
   a. 10%   b. 20%   c. 30%

6. Currently, over _____ of North Americans die of cardiovascular disease.
   a. 20%   b. 40%   c. 60%

7. Today, a 65-year-old U.S. male can expect to live _____ years longer than his counterpart did in 1900.
   a. 4   b. 8   c. 12

8. At the turn of the century around _____ of Americans died from coronary heart disease and stroke.
   a. under 10%   b. 20%   c. 30%

9. It has been estimated that up to _____ of heart attacks before age 65 could be prevented by lifestyle measures.
   a. 25%   b. 50%   c. 80%

10. A healthy diet would _____ my grocery bills.
    a. increase   b. not affect   c. decrease

11. Since 1945, adult onset diabetes (Type 2) in the U.S. has increased by _____.
    a. 100%   b. 300%   c. 500%   d. 700%

12. Countries with the highest per capita dairy consumption have _____ rates of osteoporosis (brittle bones).
    a. decreased   b. increased   c. about the same

13. Caffeine intake has been associated with _____.
    a. sleep disturbances   b. stomach ulcers   c. calcium loss from bones   d. all

14. _____ is the best way to build muscles.
    a. Eating more protein   b. Eating more starch   c. Exercise

15. One gram of fat contains _____ number of calories as one gram of either protein or carbohydrate.
   a. half the   b. the same   c. more than twice the

16. Which contains the most calories?
   a. 5 oz. potato   b. 5 oz. beefsteak   c. 5 oz. bread

17. Most North Americans eat _____ protein than needed.
   a. less   b. slightly more   c. two times more

18. An average piece of pie contains about _____ teaspoons of sugar.
   a. 10   b. 15   c. 20

19. Osteoporosis is promoted by _____.
   a. caffeine   b. smoking   c. high protein diet   d. all of these

20. _____ is the most important risk factor for coronary heart disease.
   a. High blood pressure   b. Smoking   c. High blood cholesterol level   d. Stress

21. An ideal, safe cholesterol level for middle-aged adults is _____.
   a. under 160 mg%   b. 160-200 mg%   c. 200-240 mg%   d. under 260 mg%

22. _____ fat poses the greatest danger in heart disease.
   a. Unsaturated   b. Saturated   c. Mono-unsaturated

23. The least amount of cholesterol is found in _____.
   a. 1 c. custard   b. 5 oz. steak   c. 5 oz. chicken   d. 4 oz. peanut butter

24. The body requires a minimum of _____ teaspoon(s) of salt per day.
   a. $\frac{1}{10}$ b. 1   c. 2

25. Most Westerners eat about _____ teaspoon(s) of salt per day.
   a. $\frac{1}{2}$ b. 1   c. 2   d. 3+

26. High fat diets are linked to which types of cancer?
   a. colon   b. breast   c. prostate   d. all of these

27. _____ of essential hypertension can be normalized through dietary means.
   a. 20%   b. 40%   c. 60%   d. 75%

28. Which food contains the most salt?
   a. cheeseburger   b. milkshake   c. apple pie   d. French fries

29. A 12 oz. soft drink averages _____ teaspoons of sugar.
   a. 1-3   b. 4-7   c. 8-10   d. over 10

30. The best way to lose weight permanently is to eat _____.
   a. more protein   b. more fat   c. more starchy foods

ANSWERS: *1-c 2-c 3-c 4-c 5-b 6-b 7-a 8-a 9-c 10-c 11-d 12-b 13-d 14-c 15-c 16-b 17-c*
18-b 19-d 20-c 21-a 22-b 23-d 24-a 25-d 26-d 27-d 28-a 29-c 30-c

Recommended Cookbooks

Of These Ye May Freely Eat—a vegetarian cookbook with more that 250 CHIP-approved recipes by JoAnn Rachor. US$3.95.

Cooking With Natural Foods—more than 450 CHIP-approved recipes by Muriel Beltz. 195 pages. US$14.95.

Eat to Your Health—a primer to CHIP-approved recipes by Shirley Venden. 187 pages. US$9.95.

Weimar Institute—NEWSTART® Lifestyle Cookbook—260 Heart-Healthy Recipes featuring Whole Plant Foods. 225 pages. US$21.95. Thomas Nelson Publishers (615-889-9000).

Resources

Audiotape Albums

*"**Diet for a New Century**"—A Smarter, Saner Choice. Learn how to Live Longer, Feel Better, Have Better Health, Save Money, and Protect the Environment. Two cassettes in a full-color album. US$17.95.

*"**Eat More for Better Health**"—Six-tape series offers solutions that can reverse hypertension, heart disease, diabetes, and obesity by attacking the causes. US$39.95.

Videotapes

*"**Better Health: New Beginnings**"—Keys to Living Longer and Feeling Better. After watching these fast-moving, motivational, and entertaining videos, you won't be the same. Tens of thousands have been helped by putting into practice Dr. Diehl's revolutionary lifestyle guidelines. This 9-part video (totaling six hours) is for those who want to feel younger and "Live with ALL their Hearts"—longer and better. Try this proven plan, and in four weeks you can change your life forever. US$75.00.

*"**To Your Health**"—The most popular video in the *Search* telecast series in 18 years! Entertaining, scientific, motivating. The ideal gift if you want to help someone to get out of hypertension, diabetes (II), heart disease, high cholesterol, and obesity. 34 minutes. US$20.00.

*Available at
Lifestyle Medicine Institute
P.O. Box 474
Loma Linda, CA 92354
909-796-7676